Family-Based Treatment in Child and Adolescent Psychiatry

Editors

MICHELLE L. RICKERBY
THOMAS A. ROESLER

CHILD AND ADOLESCENT PSYCHIATRIC CLINICS OF NORTH AMERICA

www.childpsych.theclinics.com

Consulting Editor
HARSH K. TRIVEDI

July 2015 • Volume 24 • Number 3

ELSEVIER

1600 John F. Kennedy Boulevard • Suite 1800 • Philadelphia, Pennsylvania, 19103-2899

http://www.theclinics.com

CHILD AND ADOLESCENT PSYCHIATRIC CLINICS OF NORTH AMERICA Volume 24, Number 3
July 2015 ISSN 1056-4993, ISBN-13: 978-0-323-39090-3

Editor: Joanne Husovski
Developmental Editor: Stephanie Wissler

Child and Adolescent Psychiatric Clinics of North America (ISSN 1056-4993) is published quarterly by Elsevier Inc., 360 Park Avenue South, New York, NY 10010-1710. Months of issue are January, April, July, and October. Business and Editorial Offices: 1600 John F. Kennedy Boulevard, Suite 1800, Philadelphia, PA 19103-2899. Periodicals postage paid at New York, NY and additional mailing offices. Subscription prices are $310.00 per year (US individuals), $491.00 per year (US institutions), $155.00 per year (US students), $360.00 per year (Canadian individuals), $598.00 per year (Canadian institutions), $200.00 per year (Canadian students), $430.00 per year (international individuals), $598.00 per year (international institutions), and $200.00 per year (international students). International air speed delivery is included in all *Clinics* subscription prices. All prices are subject to change without notice. **POSTMASTER:** Send address changes to *Child and Adolescent Psychiatric Clinics of North America*, Elsevier Health Sciences Division, Subscription Customer Service, 3251 Riverport Lane, Maryland Heights, MO 63043. **Customer Service: 1-800-654-2452 (U.S. and Canada); 314-447-8871 (outside U.S. and Canada). Fax: 314-447-8029. E-mail: JournalsCustomer Service-usa@elsevier.com (for print support) or journalsonlinesupport-usa@elsevier.com (for online support).**

Reprints. For copies of 100 or more of articles in this publication, please contact the Commercial Reprints Department, Elsevier Inc., 360 Park Avenue South, New York, New York 10010-1710 Tel.: 212-633-3874; Fax: 212-633-3820, E-mail: reprints@elsevier.com.

Child and Adolescent Psychiatric Clinics of North America is covered in *MEDLINE/PubMed (Index Medicus), ISI, SSCI, Research Alert, Social Search, Current Contents,* and *EMBASE/Excerpta Medica.*

Contributors

CONSULTING EDITOR

HARSH K. TRIVEDI, MD, MBA
Executive Director and Chief Medical Officer; Behavioral Health Vice Chair for Clinical Affairs; Associate Professor of Psychiatry, Vanderbilt University School of Medicine, Nashville, Tennessee

CONSULTING EDITOR EMERITUS

ANDRÉS MARTIN, MD, MPH

FOUNDING CONSULTING EDITOR

MELVIN LEWIS, MBBS, FRCPSYCH, DCH

EDITORS

MICHELLE L. RICKERBY, MD
Associate Clinical Professor, Department of Psychiatry and Human Behavior, The Alpert School of Medicine of Brown University; Psychiatric Director, Hasbro Children's Partial Hospital Program; Psychiatric Director of Child Medical/Psychiatric Services for Lifespan, Providence, Rhode Island

THOMAS A. ROESLER, MD
Professor, Department of Psychiatry and Behavioral Sciences, University of Washington School of Medicine; Medical Director, Psychiatry and Behavioral Medicine Unit, Seattle Children's Hospital, Seattle, Washington

AUTHORS

LINDSAY M. ANDERSON, MA
Department of Psychology and Neuroscience, Duke University, Durham, North Carolina

JUDITH A. COHEN, MD
Professor of Psychiatry, Allegheny General Hospital, Drexel University College of Medicine, Pittsburgh, Pennsylvania

SUSAN DICKSTEIN, PhD
Associate Professor, Departments of Psychiatry and Human Behavior and Pediatrics, Bradley Hospital/Warren Medical School of Brown University, Providence, Rhode Island

SARAH FORSBERG, PsyD
Clinical Instructor, Department of Psychiatry and Behavioral Sciences, Stanford University, Stanford, California

MARTIN E. FRANKLIN, PhD
Department of Psychiatry, University of Pennsylvania Medical School, Philadelphia, Pennsylvania

JENNIFER B. FREEMAN, PhD
Department of Psychiatry and Human Behavior, Warren Alpert Medical School of Brown University, Providence, Rhode Island

MARY A. FRISTAD, PhD, ABPP
Professor, Departments of Psychiatry and Behavioral Health, Psychology, and Nutrition; Associate Director for Research, Center for Integrative Health and Wellness, The Ohio State University, Columbus, Ohio

ERIC GOEPFERT, MD
Departments of Pediatrics and Child and Adolescent Psychiatry, Tufts Medical Center, Boston, Massachusetts

LYNN HERNANDEZ, PhD
Assistant Professor of Behavioral and Social Sciences, Center for Alcohol and Addiction Studies, Brown University School of Public Health, Providence, Rhode Island

ALLAN M. JOSEPHSON, MD
CEO, Bingham Clinic; Professor and Chief, Division of Child and Adolescent Psychiatry, Department of Pediatrics, University of Louisville School of Medicine, Louisville, Kentucky

DOUGLAS A. KRAMER, MD, MS
Emeritus Clinical Professor of Psychiatry, University of Wisconsin School of Medicine and Public Health, Madison, Wisconsin

JAMES LOCK, MD, PhD
Professor, Department of Psychiatry and Behavioral Sciences, Stanford University, Stanford, California

JULIANA MANGANELLA, BA
Research Coordinator, Division of Pain Medicine, Department of Anesthesiology, Perioperative and Pain Medicine, Boston Children's Hospital, Massachusetts

ANTHONY P. MANNARINO, PhD
Professor of Psychiatry, Allegheny General Hospital, Drexel University College of Medicine, Pittsburgh, Pennsylvania

CHRISTINA MULÉ, PhD
Departments of Pediatrics and Child and Adolescent Psychiatry, Tufts Medical Center, Boston, Massachusetts

JEFF RANDALL, PhD
Department of Psychiatry and Behavioral Sciences, Family Services Research Center, Medical University of South Carolina, Charleston, South Carolina

MICHELLE L. RICKERBY, MD
Associate Clinical Professor, Department of Psychiatry and Human Behavior, The Alpert School of Medicine of Brown University; Psychiatric Director, Hasbro Children's Partial Hospital Program, Providence, Rhode Island

ANA MARIA RODRIGUEZ, MS
Intervention Specialist, Center for Alcohol and Addiction Studies, Brown University School of Public Health, Providence, Rhode Island

THOMAS A. ROESLER, MD
Professor, Department of Psychiatry and Behavioral Sciences, University of Washington School of Medicine; Medical Director, Psychiatry and Behavioral Medicine Unit, Seattle Children's Hospital, Seattle, Washington

JEFFREY J. SAPYTA, PhD
Department of Psychiatry and Behavioral Sciences, Duke University School of Medicine, Durham, North Carolina

JOHN SARGENT, MD
Professor of Psychiatry and Pediatrics, Tufts School of Medicine; Chief of Child Psychiatry Division, Department of Psychiatry, Tufts Medical Center, Boston, Massachusetts

NEHA SHARMA, DO
Assistant Professor of Psychiatry, Tufts School of Medicine; Program Director of Child Psychiatry Fellowship, Department of Psychiatry, Tufts Medical Center, Boston, Massachusetts

CHRISTINE B. SIEBERG, PhD
Staff Psychologist, Pain Treatment Service, Boston Children's Hospital; Assistant Professor of Psychology, Department of Psychiatry, Harvard Medical School, Massachusetts

MATTHEW SIEGEL, MD
Maine Medical Center Research Institute, Scarborough, Maine

ANTHONY SPIRITO, PhD, ABPP
Professor and Vice Chair, Division of Clinical Psychology, Department of Psychiatry and Human Behavior, Alpert Medical School of Brown University, Providence, Rhode Island

CYNTHIA CUPIT SWENSON, PhD
Department of Psychiatry and Behavioral Sciences, Family Services Research Center, Medical University of South Carolina, Charleston, South Carolina

ZACHARY VISCO, BA
Departments of Pediatrics and Child and Adolescent Psychiatry, Tufts Medical Center, Boston, Massachusetts

ERIK VON HAHN, MD
Departments of Pediatrics and Child and Adolescent Psychiatry, Tufts Medical Center, Boston, Massachusetts

ANDREA S. YOUNG, PhD
Department of Psychiatry and Behavioral Health, The Ohio State University Wexner Medical Center, Columbus, Ohio

KRISTYN ZAJAC, PhD
Department of Psychiatry and Behavioral Sciences, Family Services Research Center, Medical University of South Carolina, Charleston, South Carolina

Contents

> From early twentieth century social reform movements emerged the ingredients for both child and family psychiatry. Both psychiatries that involve children, parents, and families began in child guidance clinics. Post–World War II intellectual creativity provided the epistemological framework for treating families. Eleven founders (1950–1969) led the development of family psychiatry. Child and family psychiatrists disagreed over the issues of individual and family group dynamics. Over the past 25 years the emerging sciences of interaction, in the context of the Primate Social Organ System (PSOS), have produced the evidence for the family being the entity of treatment in psychiatry.

> For many, family therapy refers to sessions in which all family members are present. Yet in contemporary psychiatry there are many ways to work with families in addition to this classic concept. This article proposes *family intervention* as an encompassing term for a new family paradigm in child and adolescent psychiatry. Developmental psychopathology is a guiding principle of this paradigm. A full range of ways to work with families clinically is described with clinical examples.

> This article provides updated information about evidence-based family interventions for child and adolescent mental health issues. The article reviews randomized controlled trials for family-based interventions carried out over the last 15 years. The studies were selected from an evidence-based clearinghouse search for family therapy, and specific child and adolescent psychiatric disorders. It is hoped this review guides clinical treatment and encourages clinicians to consider family involvement in treatment. This is specifically necessary when there is a limited response to psychopharmacologic and individual or group psychotherapy treatment.

of pediatric OCD. Special attention is given to relevant contextual family processes that influence symptom presentation, current empirical support for family-based treatment, and the clinical application of family-based cognitive-behavioral therapy. Case vignettes illustrate important clinical considerations for providers.

Trauma-focused cognitive behavioral therapy (TF-CBT) is a family-focused treatment in which parents or caregivers participate equally with their traumatized child or adolescent. TF-CBT is a components-based and phase-based treatment that emphasizes proportionality and incorporates gradual exposure into each component. Child and parent receive all TF-CBT components in parallel individual sessions that enhance skills to help the child recognize and regulate trauma responses, express thoughts and feelings about the child's trauma experiences and master avoidance of trauma memories and reminders. Parental participation significantly enhances the beneficial impact of TF-CBT for traumatized children.

The increasing prevalence of autism spectrum disorder (ASD), the severity of impairment, and its impact on systems are a source of ever-growing concern. This article (1) describes briefly the spectrum of ASD and its treatments; (2) discusses the impact that ASD has on the individual, family, and external environment; and (3) discusses the application of family therapy principles in order to meet the needs of children and families affected by ASD. Illustrative case examples are presented.

Research has shown that a lack of parental involvement in their children's activities predicts initiation and escalation of substance use. Parental monitoring and supervision, parent-child communication including communication regarding beliefs and disapproval of substance use, positive parenting, and family management strategies, have been shown to protect against adolescent substance abuse and related problems. Family and parenting approaches to preventing and intervening on adolescent substance abuse have received support in the literature. This article discusses the theoretical foundations as well as the application of the Family Check-up, a brief, family-based intervention for adolescent substance use.

Externalizing problems are multidetermined and related to individual, family, peer, school, and community risk factors. Multisystemic therapy (MST) was originally developed to address these risk factors among youth with serious conduct problems who are at-risk for out-of-home placement. Several decades of research have established MST as an evidence-based intervention for adolescents with serious clinical problems, including serious offending, delinquency, substance abuse, and parental physical abuse and neglect. This article presents an overview of the clinical procedures and evidence base of MST for externalizing problems as well as 2 adaptations: MST for Substance Abuse and MST for Child Abuse and Neglect.

Best-practice guidelines for the treatment of child and adolescent eating disorders recommend the inclusion of parents. Family-based treatment (FBT) posits that families are not only important in supporting their children but are critical change agents in the recovery process. As originally developed for anorexia nervosa, parents take a central role in managing and disrupting eating disorder symptoms. The most evidence-based treatment model for adolescent anorexia nervosa, FBT has also recently been found to be useful in the treatment of adolescent bulimia nervosa. This article provides a summary of the theoretic model, evidence base, and application of FBT.

Whether a child has to endure a procedure that incurs acute pain or a child has chronic pain, the impact on the family, especially parents, can be profound. Parents need to be active members of their child's health care team; however, they are often ill equipped to cope with either acute pain stressors or longstanding chronic pain in their children. This article provides an overview of acute and chronic pain, the impact of parent factors on pediatric pain, parental assessments of parent functioning, and parent-based interventions for pediatric pain management. Case examples are used to illustrate the treatments presented.

CHILD AND ADOLESCENT PSYCHIATRIC CLINICS

CHILD AND ADOLESCENT PSYCHIATRIC CLINICS

FORTHCOMING ISSUES

October 2015
Global Mental Health
Ronald T. Joshi and Lisa M. Cullins,
Editors

January 2016
Adjudicated Youth
Harshan A. Zerby, Editor

April 2016
Prevention in Child Mental Wellness:
Improving Population Health
Aradhana Bela Sood and
James T. Hudziak, Editors

RECENT ISSUES

April 2015
School Mental Health
Margaret M. Benningfield and
Sharon Hoover Stephan, Editors

January 2015
Top Topics in Child and Adolescent
Psychiatry
Harsh K. Trivedi, Editor

October 2014
ADHD: Non-Pharmacologic Interventions
Stephen V. Faraone and
Kevin M. Antshel, Editors

Preface

An Introduction to Family-Based Treatment in Child Psychiatry

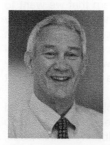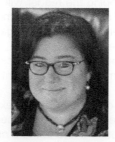

Thomas A. Roesler, MD   Michelle L. Rickerby, MD
Editors

This issue of *Child and Adolescent Psychiatric Clinics of North America* had its origins in the discussions over the past few years of the Committee on the Family of the American Academy of Child and Adolescent Psychiatry. As a group the members of the committee have reflected on how enormous the range and depth of 'biopsychosocial' knowledge the modern child psychiatrist needs to master including neurobiology, genetics, psychopharmacology, and psychological processes in individuals, families, and social groups. Although we had no reason to believe our colleagues fundamentally disagreed with us, we felt there could be a lack of awareness by some regarding the depth and breadth of evidence to support family-based interventions in child psychiatry. We felt that given the rapid advances in psychopharmacologic therapies, the application of manualized cognitive behavioral therapy (CBT) and dialectical behavior therapy approaches targeting individual children, and even the introduction of the DSM V, that the balance has shifted away from what traditionally was meant by the term, "well-trained child psychiatrist."

We also noted the time might be right for a review of the evidence supporting family-based treatments. We were all aware that advances in neuropsychiatry were spotlighting the epigenetic effects of relationship contexts in the development of both mental health disorders and physical illnesses. We could point to the "family-centered care" initiatives present in almost all the medical institutions in which we practiced. We had the Federal government make it national policy that medical and mental health care be delivered in settings that emphasized prevention and health maintenance rather than primarily symptom resolution. We could read articles in major newspapers about the overuse of psychoactive medicine in children.

Child Adolesc Psychiatric Clin N Am 24 (2015) xiii–xv
http://dx.doi.org/10.1016/j.chc.2015.03.002
1056-4993/15/$ – see front matter © 2015 Published by Elsevier Inc.

These broad-based currents swirling around us made it seem that the pendulum was truly swinging back from a reductionistic view of a symptom in a child to a more balanced view of a symptom in a child existing in a family and cultural context.

We have avoided the term "family therapy" in the title of this issue. We were partially influenced by the fact that no clear definition exists for the term. Many forms of family treatments use the term and actually refer to substantially different things. Rather, we have used "family-based treatment," hoping the reader will discern that we want to include a wide variety of practice that all starts from the premise that children typically exist in families and that to attempt to help them while disregarding the environment in which they live is often ineffective. See both Kramer in the opening article and Josephson in the second article to understand the difference between family therapy as a specific treatment modality and family-based treatment as a way to think about children.

A similar confusion surrounds the use of other terms. For example, "family-centered care" has many definitions. In some cases, the term family-centered care has come to mean "the family is always right." The editors and authors contributing to this issue, taken together, can claim many hundreds of years working with families. We are fully aware of the tasks required of families as they go about the work of surviving economically, providing for mutual support, and helping individual family members, both adults and children, to grow in developmentally appropriate ways. But the families are the first to tell us that what they do, and believe, and feel are not always conducive to the outcomes they desire. They come with symptoms or problems or goals and ask us to help with those things primarily by helping them do, or believe, or feel something different from what they were trying before. Recognizing that many forms of treatment for many different conditions can begin with putting the family first is not the same as saying that whatever the family wants or has been doing is truly best for the individual with the presenting symptom or the family as a whole.

This issue is divided into two parts. The first part includes articles of a more general nature: the history of the field; some guidelines for family assessment; a review of evidence-based studies; some thoughts about young children in families; and finishes with an example of a training program that prepares child psychiatrists for family-based child psychiatry. The second part features descriptions of family-based treatments of common child psychiatric conditions written by researchers and clinicians who have contributed significantly to the field of child psychiatry over the past decade. Here one finds, among the list of topics, Cohen and Mannarino outlining their well-researched trauma-focused CBT for traumatized children, and Forsberg and Lock writing about treatment of teenagers with eating disorders.

Our aim in creating this edition was to develop a resource that would be equally valuable to trainees as well as to practicing child psychiatrists from a broad range of experience and practice settings. In addition, we had an eye to providing a cross-disciplinary resource focused on the broad range of family based integrated care as applied to common psychiatric diagnoses and as an overarching model for all treatment. Our hope is for the reader to agree with us that the "well trained child psychiatrist," while treating the child, will always have the family in view. And, that the coordination of care across disciplines can operate like a healthy functioning family.

Thomas A. Roesler, MD
Department of Psychiatry and Behavioral Sciences
University of Washington School of Medicine
Seattle, WA 98105, USA

Psychiatry and Behavioral Medicine Unit
Seattle Children's Hospital
Seattle, WA, USA

Michelle L. Rickerby, MD
Hasbro Partial Hospital Program
Hasbro Children's Hospital
593 Eddy Street, Providence, RI 02903, USA

E-mail addresses:
troesler88@gmail.com (T.A. Roesler)
MRickerby@Lifespan.org (M.L. Rickerby)

History of Family Psychiatry

From the Social Reform Era to the Primate Social Organ System

Douglas A. Kramer, MD, MS

KEYWORDS

- Family • Family therapy • Family intervention • Family psychiatry
- Biological psychiatry • Comprehensive biological treatment
- Natural healing mechanisms • Primate Social Organ System • PSOS

KEY POINTS

- Child psychiatry and family psychiatry emerged in the context of the social reform movements of the early twentieth century.
- Child psychiatry and family psychiatry began in the child guidance clinics in the United States and Great Britain.
- In order of the first family publications, the founders of family psychiatry include Nathan Ackerman, Gregory Bateson, Carl Whitaker, Don Jackson, Lyman Wynne, Jay Haley, Virginia Satir, Ivan Boszormenyi-Nagy, Salvador Minuchin, Murray Bowen, and John Bowlby.
- With the emergence of family psychiatry (circa 1950), the relationship between child psychiatry and family psychiatry has evolved from estrangement, to impasse, to détente, and finally to synthesis.
- The primate brain evolved under selection pressure for social competence.
- The biopsychosocial family is the extended family social group.
- The sciences of interaction are (1) nonlinear brain dynamics, (2) gene-environment interaction, and (3) epigenetics, and these make obsolete current diagnostic and treatment frameworks in psychiatry.
- The organ system in psychiatry is the Primate Social Organ System (PSOS), consisting of all the brains typically in relationship to each other.

OVERVIEW

A lack of congruence in nomenclature regarding psychiatrists who treat families has existed for more than 6 decades. Almost universally, and definitely into the second half of the twentieth century, child psychiatrists had only so-called therapies to offer patients. Psychoanalytically derived treatments were available, as well as other

Disclosures: None.
Department of Psychiatry, University of Wisconsin School of Medicine and Public Health, 6001 Research Park Boulevard, Madison, WI 53719, USA
E-mail address: dakrame1@wisc.edu

Child Adolesc Psychiatric Clin N Am 24 (2015) 439–455
http://dx.doi.org/10.1016/j.chc.2015.02.001
1056-4993/15/$ – see front matter © 2015 Elsevier Inc. All rights reserved.

childpsych.theclinics.com

therapies for children and adolescents related to conflicts; adaptations; defenses; parent-child relationships; social relationships; learning; and psychological, psychosocial, and psychosexual development.[1] Psychiatrists who treated children and adolescents using therapies called themselves child psychiatrists. Psychiatrists who treated families using therapies called themselves family therapists.

This distinction had, and continues to have, many determinants. Child psychiatry had reached a degree of maturity as a profession by the time psychiatrists and other mental health professionals started treating families, around or just before 1950.[2] Family psychiatry was in a stage of development analogous to Erikson's "identity versus role confusion." The family therapy field did not know whether its practitioners did interviews with whole families, (1) simply to gather information thoroughly and efficiently; (2) as a context within which to treat individuals or pairs of individuals (eg, the mother-child dyad); or (3) to treat an organism greater than the sum of its parts, the parts being all of the individuals and relationships in the family, and the whole being an emergent property of that complex organism.[3]

There were additional issues for the field to resolve, including (1) whether the term "family" described a therapy technique or a patient entity; (2) whether family therapy was a medical or a psychosocial therapy; and (3) whether a therapy other than one based on individual psychodynamics could be considered psychiatric.

Nomenclature issues can never be resolved until the entity being named is fully understood. This article reviews the history of the treatment of families in psychiatry, and concludes that the correct name of the field is *family psychiatry*. An interesting consideration in the age of biological psychiatry is whether family psychiatry just might be the only truly comprehensive biological psychiatry?[4-7]

SOCIAL REFORM MOVEMENTS

Social reform movements, and the birth of organizations and institutions devoted to the mental health of children and families, in the first quarter of the twentieth century planted the seeds and fertilized the soil for the birth of child psychiatry and family psychiatry. The reform movements included the Settlement Movement, Mental Hygiene Movement, Child Guidance Movement, The Commonwealth Fund, Juvenile Courts, and American Orthopsychiatric Association. The vibrancy of these movements, led by a combination of citizen activists, middle-class and upper-class reformers, and concerned professionals, grew even during World War I, the Great Pandemic, Prohibition, Black Tuesday, the Great Depression, and the approaching World War II. There existed unstoppable concern for children, women, and families at all levels of society.

Mental Hygiene Movement

Founded in New York City in 1909, the National Committee for Mental Hygiene (NCMH) worked, "to humanize the public attitude towards those afflicted with mental disease."[8] The organizers of the NCMH included Adolph Meyer, William James, and Clifford W. Beers, a Yale-educated, upper-class man who was hospitalized several times for mental illness. Beers' book about experiences in psychiatric facilities, *A Mind That Found Itself,* published in 1908, helped catalyze the formation of the Committee, and aided in solicitation of funds from other well-to-do families and Ivy League friends.[9]

Additional financial support for the NCMH was provided by The Commonwealth Fund. The latter was established in 1918 by Anna M. Harkness "to do something for the welfare of mankind." The Fund developed a Five Year Program for the Prevention of Delinquency (1921), devoted to severe difficulties of "personality and behavior" in children predisposed to delinquency.[10] The establishment of the Five Year Program recognized the approach among professionals caring for children fragmented the child.

In planning the work of the division it was early recognized that in spite of the progress made in various phases of child health and child welfare, these activities to date were uncoordinated, that each group was only taking a fractional interest in the child and treating him either as a mind to be educated, a physical organism to be safeguarded or an offender to be disciplined.[8]

Child Guidance Movement

The idea leading to the first child guidance clinic came from reform-minded citizens in Chicago. They were associated with Hull House, a "settlement house," founded by Jane Addams. It was one of more than 400 such communities in the United States working to alleviate difficulties associated with poverty. The settlement houses provided education, daycare, medical care, and other services in a communal living arrangement of low-income residents and middle-class volunteers.

Similar to the spark provided by Clifford Beers in 1908 leading to the formation of the NCMH, Mrs Ethel Dummer of Chicago in 1909 became the catalyst for the child guidance movement. She was a volunteer at Hull House, a member of the Board of the Juvenile Protective Association, and a frequent visitor to Cook County Juvenile Court, which was led by the reformist judge, Merritt W. Pinckney. Her donation funded the study and treatment of delinquency for 5 years.[11]

Mrs Dummer's philanthropy led to the founding of the Juvenile Psychopathic Institute (1909), subsequently renamed the Psychopathic Clinic of the Juvenile Court (1914), Illinois Juvenile Psychopathic Institute (1917), Illinois Institute for Juvenile Research, and eventually the Institute for Juvenile Research (1920), later known simply as IJR. The Juvenile Psychopathic Institute was the first child guidance clinic and the model for all subsequent child guidance clinics.

The First Child and Adolescent Psychiatrist

Dr William Healy outlined the plan for this new institute, and thus for the child guidance movement. The plan included "a careful physical examination, special school reports from teachers, interviews with parents and relatives to ascertain 'heredity, developmental personality peculiarities, family relationships, and much else.'"[11] Dr Healy was a British-born neurologist practicing at the Chicago Polyclinic before becoming Medical Director of the Juvenile Psychopathic Institute.

In 1915, Dr Healy published, *The Individual Delinquent,* his analysis of more than 800 case studies completed at the Juvenile Psychopathic Clinic.[12] Levy places *The Individual Delinquent* and Healy's work in historical context: "The book had an amazing influence on legal procedures, on the fields of sociology, anthropology, psychology, and especially psychiatry. The fact that the child guidance movement started in the field of delinquency made necessary the utilization of a team—psychologist, psychiatrist, and social worker."[11]

Was William Healy the first child and adolescent psychiatrist? Julius B. Richmond, pediatrician, Project Head Start originator, and Surgeon General, implies as much: "A Chicago physician, Dr William Healy, in 1909 organized the first child guidance clinic in the world... establishment of this clinic under medical auspices served as a stimulus for the development of child psychiatry as a discipline."[13]

American Orthopsychiatric Association

The American Orthopsychiatric Association (Ortho) was founded in 1923 by 9 psychiatrists, including Herman Adler, V. V. Anderson, Bernard Glueck, William Healy, Arnold Jacoby, David Levy, Lawson Lowery, Karl Menninger, and George Stevenson. Many of the psychiatrists, physicians, and other professionals who were active in the child guidance movement, were active in Ortho (an organization not restricted to physicians), paralleling the team approach practiced in child guidance clinics. The *American Journal of Orthopsychiatry* began publication in 1930.

ORIGIN OF FAMILY PSYCHIATRY

The primary loci for treatment of children for approximately 50 years were the child guidance clinics. Psychiatrists, pediatricians, and neurologists, working in teams with psychologists and social workers, applied the formula devised by William Healy in 1908. The system of child guidance clinics was totally decentralized for almost 4 decades. The individual child guidance clinics had working relationships with juvenile courts and social service agencies in their communities.

There were relationships among the professionals with the NCMH, The Commonwealth Fund, and Ortho, and relationships among the physicians with the American Psychiatric Association (APA) and the American Academy of Pediatrics (AAP). The literature hints at some uncertainty as to the primary specialty (psychiatry or pediatrics) with which such a physician, addressing the mental health needs of children and adolescents, might be identified. The totally decentralized system of child guidance clinics became more centralized in 1948 when 54 clinics affiliated with the new American Association of Psychiatric Clinics for Children (AAPCC), 39 years after the Juvenile Psychopathic Institute opened its doors.

Early Landscape of Family Psychiatry

Movements begin and proliferate when an idea makes so much sense in a culture that it has multiple originations. Family probably was on the minds of physicians when house calls, and giving birth at home, were common. With the heightened interest in children and adolescents early in the twentieth century, it is reasonable that parents might have come to the minds of professionals, which they did because the first, and all subsequent, child guidance clinics included parents in their diagnostic and treatment efforts.

The intellectual and scientific climate coincident with the emergence of family psychiatry was exciting, especially studies of behavior and the development of hypotheses applicable to *Homo sapiens*. **Table 1** lists important intellectual events coincident with the origins of family psychiatry.

Table 1
Intellectual landscape: 1946 to 1953

Date	Science	Authors	Publication, Film, or Event
1946	Cybernetics	Warren McCulloch	First Josiah Macy Cybernetics Conference[14]
1946	Psychiatry	William Menninger	Group for the Advancement of Psychiatry[15]
1949	Ecology	Aldo Leopold	A Sand County Almanac[16]
1951	Ethology	Niko Tinbergen	The Study of Instinct[17]
1951	Communication	Jurgen Ruesch & Gregory Bateson	Communication: The Social Matrix of Psychiatry[18]
1953	Attachment	John Bowlby & James Robertson	A Two-Year Old Goes to the Hospital[19]
1953	Psychotherapy	Carl A. Whitaker & Thomas P. Malone	The Roots of Psychotherapy[20]

Family Psychiatry Movement

My own understanding of family therapy, which I always understood to be family psychiatry, because it seemed mostly practiced by psychiatrists, began in 1975, my first year of psychiatry residency. My teachers and supervisors included Carl Whitaker, MD,[21] David Keith, MD,[22] Jack Westman, MD,[23] Augustus Napier, PhD,[24] Richard Anderson, MD,[25] and Jack P. Hailman, PhD.[26] My understanding of the history of family psychiatry is unavoidably influenced by my relationships and experience.

Origins of the Idea: Nathan W. Ackerman (1908–1971)

After a rotating internship and an assistant residency in neurology at Montefiore Hospital (1933–1935), Ackerman did a neuropsychiatry residency at Menninger Clinic and Sanitarium (1935–1936). He joined the staff of Menninger Clinic in 1936, becoming Assistant Medical Director of Southard School (1936–1937), probably the Menninger Child Guidance Clinic.[27] He returned to New York City in 1937 where he founded the Family Institute in 1960 (renamed The Ackerman Institute for the Family following his death in 1971), and cofounded the journal Family Process with Jay Haley (1961).

The family psychiatry movement had multiple loci of origination and multiple parents, speaking multiple languages, with much of the history never recorded. Just as with child psychiatry, the child guidance clinics were prominent in the early conceptions of family psychiatry. However, there was not a single father or mother, a William Healy, of family psychiatry. If there were one, he would be Nathan Ackerman. In a 1970 presentation, published posthumously in 1972, Ackerman referred to the idea of family psychiatry as "my primary interest in the psychiatry of the whole family."[28]

Based on his own writing, including his insistence on developing a theory of family therapy before attempting to treat a family, he almost certainly was not the first psychiatrist to treat whole families. However, his ability to define the goal of family diagnoses and family group treatment at professional meetings and in print,[2,29] and his openness regarding the difficulties in transitioning from individual to family group psychodynamics, were a vital contribution to family psychiatry.

In his first publication on the treatment of families (1950), Ackerman and Sobel[2] highlight the family oriented approach in child guidance clinics. They seem to say that nowhere were whole families being treated.

Accordingly, we believe that the treatment of the young child should begin with the treatment of the family group. However, we find ourselves confronted with the fact that, up to the present time, no adequate criteria for family disturbances, as group disturbances, have been found. Until such criteria are formulated so that we may describe (and later classify) such family disturbances, we have no frame of reference for the treatment of families as groups, despite the claims of many child guidance clinics to the contrary. Although the trends in child guidance are toward family orientation, the child and the mother, but not the family, are treated. We do not know whether it is possible to treat families as groups. Perhaps it is not possible.[2]

In Ackerman's final statement about the field, he reiterates his career-long goal of developing a system of family diagnosis, and the "responsibility of conceptualizing and categorizing family types." He spoke of, "a natural behavioral phenomenon, family healing... a range of self-healing processes which occur spontaneously in family life."[28]

Origins of the Idea: Carl A. Whitaker (1912–1995)

Whitaker did his internship (1936–1937) and 1 year of residency in obstetrics and gynecology (1937–1938) at City Hospital (Bellevue) in New York City. Following psychiatry residency at Syracuse University Psychopathic Hospital (1938–1940), he trained in child psychiatry at the University of Louisville Bingham Child Guidance Clinic (1940–1941), his fellowship funded by The Commonwealth Fund. From 1941 to 1944, Whitaker was the treatment psychiatrist at Ormsby Village in Anchorage, Kentucky. Ormsby was an unfenced, cottage type, coeducational facility for approximately 300 children and adolescents committed to the Louisville and Jefferson County Children's Home.[30]

In their book, *The Roots of Psychotherapy* (1953), Whitaker and Malone[18] advocate, "the importance of treating the whole family when one member of the family undertakes psychiatric treatment." Whitaker and Malone,[20] like Ackerman and Sobel,[2] saw family treatment as facilitating both better treatment of the individual patient and the relational context in which the individual patient lived. Referring to "a fundamental principle of modern ecology," the longer version of the Whitaker and Malone principle states:

Not only are the parts of an organism so interrelated that the whole is more than the sum of its parts, but the relationships among different organisms in the bionomical field are such that the whole is more than the sum of the organisms involved. The principle has led to the recognition of the importance of treating the whole family when one member of the family undertakes psychiatric treatment. We have all seen dramatic changes occur in children, both physically and psychologically, when they are moved from one environment to another. The most striking example of the sensitive interdependence among members of a family is that seen in the case of a patient who undergoes psychiatric treatment successfully. The new-found capabilities in one member of the family upsets the total economy of the family so that the other members are precipitated into a different type of pathology or therapy, or both.[20]

From 1944 to 1946, beginning their 50-year collaboration, Whitaker and Malone used nontraditional methods of psychotherapy at Oak Ridge, Tennessee.[31] The city was established by the US Army to work on the Manhattan Project. Whitaker was Director of Psychiatry. He recruited Malone to the staff. One technique they developed, multiple therapy,[32] later became known as cotherapy, and would become a core technique in the training and practice of family psychiatry. According to Malone's son, "I think they were already seeing families at Oak Ridge and continued to do so at Emory" (Patrick T. Malone, MD, personal communication, July 13, 2014). Dr Whitaker was Chair, Emory University Department of Psychiatry (1946–1955). **Fig. 1** shows Whitaker, Malone and Richard Felder, three of the original founders of the Atlanta Psychiatric Clinic, in 1987.

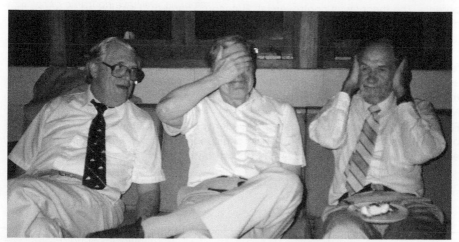

Fig. 1. Carl Whitaker, Tom Malone, and Richard Felder at a reception in Malone's home following a public presentation by Whitaker titled "Symbolic Experiential Family Therapy," at the Academy of Medicine, Atlanta, Georgia, June 12, 1987. They were attempting to pantomime, "See No Evil, Hear No Evil, Speak No Evil." (*Courtesy of* D. Kramer, MD, MS, Middleton, WI.)

Origins of the Idea: Gregory Bateson (1904–1980)

It is impossible to summarize Bateson's scholarly endeavors. Numerous books have been written describing his work, the best being the biography by David Lipset.[33] With an MA from Cambridge University in Natural Sciences and Anthropology, and 5 years as a Fellow of St John's College, he influenced during his lifetime at least 7 major areas of science, including social and cultural anthropology, evolution, ethology, communication, cybernetics, marine biology, and psychiatry. An excellent introduction to his work is *Steps to an Ecology of Mind*.[34] His best book is *Mind and Nature: A Necessary Unity*.[35] **Fig. 2** shows Gregory Bateson at a weekend seminar for a small group of psychiatry residents, including the author, in 1978.

Bateson and his colleague, social psychiatrist Jurgen Ruesch, wrote an approach to psychiatry in 1951 based on analyzing social and family relations. The preface to the 1968 edition of *Communication: The Social Matrix of Psychiatry* summarizes their formulation:

> *Notably in human systems the circuit which must be studied usually includes at least two persons... The description of a theory of communication, adapted to the human situation, and particularly to the needs of psychiatry, was the end to which this book was originally written... The convergence of physiology, ecology, and ethology—fields that study the organism's transactions with his physical and social environment—have resulted in the emergence of general systems theories of the biological sciences... Communication thus has become the social matrix of modern life.*[36]

In the first sentence of the above quotation, Ruesch and Bateson[36] establish the difference between psychiatry (and medicine) as it had always been understood, and what they brought to the discussion. Human systems involve communication (and relationship), and thus require more than 1 person; 1 person being an arbitrary distinction used in most other transactions in modern medicine.

Mental health professionals have criticized Bateson as the coauthor of the double-bind theory of schizophrenia.[37,38] The theory was seen as blaming families for schizophrenia. The theory was controversial. Bateson[39] agreed: "I am forced to agree that double bind 'theory' has contributed its share to the sufferings of those who are called (and sometimes call themselves) 'schizophrenics.'"

In reading the original 1956 publication, it is understandable that families and others felt blamed. Bateson and colleagues[37] describe patterns of relating in a manner that an anthropologist might do, operationalized those observations into 6 criteria, and theorized that they were common to schizophrenia and other human experience. Nevertheless, Bateson and Don Jackson received the 1961 Frieda Fromm-Reichmann Award from the American Academy of Psychoanalysis for their research on the "etiology, nature, or therapy of schizophrenia."[33] An interesting discussion elucidating the areas of disagreement occurred in *Psychiatric News*.[39–41]

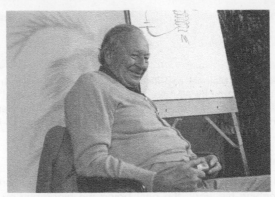

Fig. 2. Gregory Bateson at a weekend seminar in Chicago, December 2 and 3, 1978. The plan for this event had been a 2-day videotaped conversation between Bateson and Buckminster Fuller, with invited psychiatry residents as the audience. However, Fuller was unable to land in Chicago because of a snowstorm and flew on to California. Bateson landed in Indiana and made his way to the event via public transportation. (*Courtesy of* D. Kramer, MD, MS, Middleton, WI.)

Origins of the Idea: The First Family Interview: An Organic Beginning

It is impossible to know who was present at the first family therapy interview, or when and where it occurred. Perhaps a whole family arrived for an appointment at a child guidance clinic. Perhaps the social worker scheduled to see the parents had left to care for a sick child at home. Perhaps there was no one with whom to leave the younger children while the oldest saw the psychiatrist. Perhaps the psychiatrist was of a cultural background that highly valued family interactions and openness. Perhaps the psychiatrist had read or heard Ackerman or Whitaker. The psychiatrist might have considered this dilemma and said, "Why don't all of you stay, and we'll talk?"

Origins of the Idea: The Founders

Most histories of family psychiatry highlight the important thought leaders and clinicians in the early years of family psychiatry. Such an approach diminishes the grassroots origins and the organic nature of family psychiatry. As in the early days of psychoanalysis, when there were several prominent advocates shaping the field, each with a different perspective, so with family psychiatry were there a variety of proponents and associated theoretic positions. The various orientations have become less important as the field matured, akin to an adolescent experimenting with different identities while developing a single unified character. None of the identities is necessarily wrong.

Table 2 presents a list of 11 founders of family psychiatry, the order reflecting the date of the author's first family-related publication. The citation for that publication is provided. The years of birth and death are listed, as well as the founder's primary theoretic orientation.

The first family publication was determined by MEDLINE search for each name (author), and family (any field). I reviewed the title for relevance to family psychiatry. All were first authors of the articles chosen except for Gregory Bateson and Virginia Satir. Books represent first publications for 3 authors: Bateson, Whitaker, and Bowlby. There may be earlier books or chapters of which I am unaware, or articles not cataloged in MEDLINE. All of the listed individuals had several publications before the one deemed family-related (eg, Ackerman had 7 psychiatric publications shown in MEDLINE beginning in 1946, before his first family article in 1950).

Bowlby presented an interesting dilemma. His work on attachment, first published in 1953, is an important scientific foundation of child and family psychiatry.[19] It was not until 1984 that one of his cataloged articles clearly reflected a family orientation. Therefore, I chose the first volume of Attachment and Loss (1969) as a sufficiently broad treatise to qualify as family. More early contributors could certainly be added to Table 2. The goal of this list is to portray the vigorous, multidisciplinary, intellectual activity that occurred during the founding years of family psychiatry.

Origins of the Idea: Psychiatry, Child Psychiatry, and Anthropology

Of the 11 founders of family psychiatry, 8 were psychiatrists, of whom 4 were child psychiatrists (Ackerman, Whitaker, Minuchin, Bowlby). To my knowledge, Whitaker never referred to himself as a child psychiatrist, despite his training and early career experience in child psychiatry perhaps being the most extensive of any of the 11 founders. The contributions of the child psychiatrists have been the most lasting. I do not think that it is an accident that all 11 founders were born between 1904 and 1923, and thus their own childhoods, and their own families of origin, lived and developed in the environment of the social reform movements.

Table 2
Founders of family psychiatry: 1950 to 1969

Founders (First Article Reference)	First Published	Birth	Death	Theoretic Orientation
Nathan W. Ackerman, MD[2]	1950	1908	1971	Psychoanalytic
Gregory Bateson, MA[18]	1951	1904	1980	Communication - ethnology
Carl A. Whitaker, MD, MA[20]	1953	1912	1995	Experiential
Donald D. Jackson, MD[42]	1957	1920	1968	Strategic
Lyman Wynne, MD, PhD[43]	1958	1923	2007	Family communication
Jay Haley, MA[44]	1959	1923	2007	Strategic
Virginia Satir, BA[45]	1961	1916	1988	Humanistic
Ivan Boszormenyi-Nagy, MD[46]	1962	1920	2007	Intergenerational
Salvador Minuchin, MD[47]	1964	1921		Structural
Murray Bowen, MD[48]	1966	1913	1990	Family systems
John Bowlby, MD[49]	1969	1907	1990	Attachment theory - ethology

The first 3 founders' initial family publications cover a brief 4-year period. The titles are fitting for this history: "Family Diagnosis: An approach to the Preschool Child," by Ackerman and Sobel[2]; "Communication: The Social Matrix of Psychiatry," by Ruesch and Bateson[18]; and, "The Roots of Psychotherapy," by Whitaker and Malone.[20]

FAMILY PSYCHIATRY AND CHILD PSYCHIATRY

At the time family psychiatry was emerging as a new idea, in the context of a new intellectual landscape, and a new way of conceptualizing mental health and distress, the field of child psychiatry was defining itself with respect to the larger field of psychiatry. Landmark events included the APA Committee of Psychopathology of Childhood becoming the APA Section on Child Psychiatry (1943)[1]; establishment of the AAPCC (1948)[50]; formation of the AACP (1953)[1]; a ruling by the American Board of Psychiatry and Neurology (ABPN) that child guidance clinics must affiliate with approved psychiatry residency programs to train residents (1956)[50]; and creation of the Committee on Certification in Child Psychiatry by the ABPN (1959).[51]

Almost 10 years after the formation of the AACP, in an unsigned article in the first issue of the *Journal of the American Academy of Child Psychiatry* (1962) discussing the importance of an organization strictly for child psychiatrists, presumably written by the first editor, Irene Josselyn,[1] she states:

From these discussions, however, developed a conviction that just as the child is not a miniature man but an individual who through many vicissitudes will become a man, so child psychiatry, while directly related to the field of adult psychiatry as well as to other disciplines, is a specialty in itself.[1]

Josselyn's statement reflects, in my opinion, ambivalence about the path taken by organized child psychiatry. The field could not be "a specialty in itself" while at the same time being an official subspecialty of psychiatry, and historically and organizationally descended from the APA and the AAPCC. In contrast, AAP was entirely separate from the American College of Physicians; pediatricians and internal medicine specialists had separate professional organizations and separate certification boards. It is surprising that an organization whose first practitioner was a neurologist (William Healy), second practitioner a psychiatrist (George Gardner),[52] and the third a pediatrician (Julius Richmond)[12] would be so certain of its pedigree with "adult psychiatry."

Child Psychiatry and Family Psychiatry: A Complicated Relationship

On the first page of her history of AACP, Josselyn[1] hints at the necessity for an organization only for child psychiatrists despite their ongoing participation in Ortho. I suspect there are things she did not say. However, an unintended consequence of the decision was a tendency toward a cultural division between child and family psychiatrists.

The birth of a new psychiatric organization inevitably raises the question as to why, with those already in existence, an additional organization is necessary... It was probably chiefly the experiences in the Orthopsychiatric Association, in the American Association of Psychiatric Clinics for Children, and on various committees of other organizations that caused leaders in the field of child psychiatry to conclude that there was a great need for an organization specifically devoted to that field... After many discussions of the functions and limitations of those organizations, they crystallized the discontent of the child psychiatrists and formulated a solution. They contacted a group of seventeen leading child psychiatrists suggesting the possibility of an organization whose membership would be composed of child psychiatrists.[1]

I believe the decision tended to exclude most practicing child psychiatrists in the field (ie, those in the child guidance clinics, and those exploring the idea of a "psychiatry of the whole family"[28]). I believe the family-oriented psychiatrists felt at home in Ortho, and enjoyed working organizationally alongside the psychologists and social workers who were their colleagues in the clinics. They were already publishing in the *American Journal of Orthopsychiatry*, the *American Journal of Psychiatry*, and *Psychiatry: Journal for the Study of Interpersonal Processes*. Three landmark articles over 40 years (1974–2013) describe the evolving relationship between child psychiatry and family psychiatry.

Impasse (1974): The Undeclared War

Jack McDermott and Walter Char,[53] in their article, "The Undeclared War Between Child and Family Therapy," did a major service by identifying the relevant issues:

> *A good part of the problem may rest with our own specialty of child psychiatry, which seems to have been reluctant to accept a major ongoing involvement and identification with the development of the family therapy movement. Our textbooks often do not even list family therapy as a treatment modality for children. Our child psychiatry journals have pathetically few articles on work with total families.*[53]

They suggest the differences included the "family therapy movement, incorporating a strong social science element, seemed to become decidedly anti-medical,"[53] and a real or perceived desire within the family therapy community "to avoid completely individual dynamic and diagnostic terminology."[53] McDermott and Char[53] were certainly prescient. Schowalter[50] reviewed 50 years (1944–1994) of child and adolescent psychiatry in 16 pages, mentioning "family" only 5 times, and "family therapy" just twice. The only family psychiatrist named is Minuchin, with a brief uncomplimentary description, "who developed a combative and assertive style that briefly attracted many adherents."[50]

Détente (1988): Compare and Contrast

David Keith, Jack Westman, and Carl Whitaker were colleagues at the University of Wisconsin. They trained in child psychiatry in 3 different eras. In their article, they compare and contrast child psychiatry and family therapy. Whitaker's training and career are reviewed earlier. Westman trained in a psychoanalytically oriented program at the University of Michigan. Keith trained with both Westman and Whitaker but affiliated primarily with Whitaker. They describe the main differences as 2-fold: (1) is family therapy a therapeutic method or a field of practice? (2) Is the patient an individual family member, or the family as a whole?[54]

For child psychiatrists, family therapy is one of several therapeutic methods used; for family therapists it is a field of practice, a profession. For child psychiatrists, the patient is the individual family member, the treatment encompassing multisystem levels (eg, individual, family, organizational, and societal). For family therapists, the family system is the patient, the family being a "synergistic system whose whole is greater than the sum of its parts."[54]

Synthesis (2013): A Developmental Psychodynamic Therapy

Josephson's[55] 2013 article, "Family Intervention as a Developmental Psychodynamic Therapy," is a major contribution and reflects an emerging synthesis in the treatment of families. He returns to the traditional basic science of child psychiatry: child and adolescent development. He proposes the emerging discipline, developmental psychopathology, as a nontheoretic window into cause and pathogenesis. He echoes Westman's perspective,[54] the treatment including "multiple levels of analysis, from the molecular to the cultural." He views development as "the result of continual interplay between individual (developmental) and extraindividual (family) contexts."[55]

Josephson's definition of *family intervention* states, "Family intervention is defined as a coordinated set of clinical practices that alters family interaction, family environment, and parental executive functioning and, in doing so, optimizes the development of all family members."[55]

He prefers "family intervention" to "family therapy." He notes that family intervention reflects a maturation of the field beyond that of the disparate schools of family therapy. Reminiscent of both Ackerman,[28] and Whitaker and Malone,[20] his intervention, developmental psychodynamic therapy, is consistent with the natural healing mechanisms both hypothesized to be the targets of psychotherapy. Ruesch and Bateson,[36] their minimal unit of study being at least 2 persons, would likely agree with Josephson's conclusion: "What goes on between individuals affects what goes on within individuals."[55]

FAMILY PSYCHIATRY
Definition of Patient

For treatment purposes, the patient is the vehicle for achieving health, a more important consideration heuristically than the vehicle considered to be disordered. An infection requiring intravenous antibiotics requires a circulatory system for delivery, an immune system for healing, and an endocrine system for responding to acute stress. The whole-patient concept is about the entity receiving care, not about the cause or locus of the disorder.

In the *Psychiatric News* discussion about double-bind theory, Bateson's[39] response included the following (italics added), "What I will not agree to is the maltreatment of language, which would separate psychosis from the remainder of the vast spectrum of human antics–both greatness and misery. *Nor will I agree to that monstrous premise of medieval epistemology that would separate 'mind' from 'body.'*"[39]

Separating person from family is equivalent to separating mind from body, with the same unhealthy result. The other preeminent twentieth century Renaissance person (in addition to Bateson), neuroscientist Walter J. Freeman, III, agrees. He attributes the philosophic foundation on which the science of nonlinear brain dynamics rests to "one of its originators," Thomas Aquinas (1225–1274): "The core concept of intention in Aquinas is the inviolable unity of mind, brain and body."[56] In his book, *Societies of Brains,* Freeman addresses the brain and family:

> The problem is not information overload. There is always too much information. It is the misdirected search for meaning. In this they neglect the most important function of brains, which is to interact with each other to form families and societies... Meaning arises in social relations.[57]

Definitions of Family

Ackerman/Murdock definition
Ackerman[29] addresses the definition of family, insisting that it recognize production of offspring. He settles on Murdock's[58] (1949):

> The family is a social group characterized by common residence, economic cooperation and reproduction. It includes adults of both sexes, at least two of whom maintain a socially approved sexual relationship, and one or more children, own or adopted, of the sexually cohabiting adults. The vital functions of the family are sexual, economic, reproductive, and educational.[58]

Josephson definition

Josephson[55] defines family as follows (2013):

> The term "family" refers to those who have regular interaction with its children and assume the responsibility of meeting their developmental and emotional needs. It implies biological, affective, and legal bonds occurring together or separately.[55]

Kramer definition

When discussing the name of the entity to be treated, I prefer the extended family social group, the term used for all primate families (2008):

> The extended family social group: The default social condition among chimpanzees, bonobos, and primitive human groups is a community wherein most individuals are related to each other genetically or through mating and parental care. As hunting, gathering, and surviving enemies and predators occurred at this level of social organization, these human groups were subject to natural selection.[7]

Primate Social Organ System (PSOS)

Organ system concept

Medical education and practice is based on the concept of the organ system (eg, the gastrointestinal, cardiovascular, reproductive systems, etc). Attention to the organ system concept maintains intellectual integrity regarding the anatomy, physiology, development, function, and evolution of the entity being addressed. What is the organ system of interest to psychiatry? Presumably, the organ of interest is the brain. What composes the organ system to which the brain belongs?

Social brain concept

For primates, particularly the great apes, virtually the entire evolution reflects selection pressure for social competence.[59] The primate brain is a social brain primarily.[60,61] Social competence includes (1) the ability to categorize social stimuli, including vocal and nonvocal communication; (2) recognize kin and non-kin; (3) understand dominance hierarchies; (4) engage in courtship and mating behavior; (5) form alliances; (6) resolve conflict; (7) cooperate in predator vigilance and defense; (8) cooperate in foraging and hunting; (9) engage in deception; and (10) participate in social learning.[62,63]

Primate social organ system concept

An organ system for a social organ must, by definition, include other social organs (ie, other brains). One brain cannot evolve in isolation from other brains. Social organs, by necessity, interact just as fluidly as the liver and pancreas or the heart and lungs. The science of the last 25 years is consistent with the philosophies of Ackerman, Bateson, and Whitaker. The Primate Social Organ System (PSOS) is thus the organ system of interest to psychiatrists.[64,65] The PSOS is the application of the organ system concept to Walter J. Freeman's, "societies of brains."[57] The science of attachment, around which Bowlby suggested the term, developmental psychiatry,[66] demands a minimum of 2 persons. It is an artificial distinction that the organs in this organ system are located in separate individuals, an irrelevant distinction biologically. It would only be relevant in a reductionistic system. Relating, which is the function of primate brains, is not reducible.

SUMMARY
The Sciences of Interaction

During the preceding quarter century, the sciences of interaction have been extraordinarily productive. These sciences include nonlinear brain dynamics,[67–69] gene-environment interaction,[70–74] and epigenetics.[75,76]

As early as 1991, Freeman's lifetime work on nonlinear brain dynamics, or brain-environment interaction (BxE), showed that the brain (1) actively and intentionally tests the environment, (2) encodes information as a whole, (3) changes electroneurophysiologically (ie, anatomically) with each learning event, and (4) remains unchanged anatomically until a new learning event occurs.

Gene-environment interaction (GxE) is the theoretical foundation of ontogeny. In recent years, Moffitt, Caspi, Suomi, Wynne, and others have shown that offspring phenotype can be predicted from known parental phenotype, known environment, and known interaction. In some instances, the specific alleles involved have been identified.

Weaver and colleagues[75] changed entire the understanding of genetics and heredity in 2004 with "Epigenetic Programming by Maternal Behavior." In their model, maternal characteristics are transferred to offspring nongenetically, but biologically, by way of maternal behavior, through a process called *epigenetics*, which is a fundamental GxE mechanism. Cross-fostering at birth to a mother with an identical genotype, but a different phenotype, results in offspring characteristic of the foster mother.

The Thesis

The sciences of interaction, in the context of the PSOS, make obsolete all prior theories of psychiatric etiology, all prior diagnostic classifications, and all prior underpinnings of prevention and treatment strategies in psychiatry. Furthermore, the findings from the sciences of interaction are consistent with the observations, theories, and hypotheses of Ackerman, Bateson, Whitaker, Bowlby, and the other founders of family psychiatry. It all began a century ago in the context of the social reform movements of the early 20th century, and in the child guidance clinics, where for the first time children, parents, and families were treated in a coordinated fashion by teams of child mental health professionals. In conclusion, the Primate Social Organ System (PSOS) involves all of the brains that are typically in relationship, ie, the brains of each extended family social group. Thus, the patient in psychiatry is always the family, especially in a psychiatry that calls itself biological.[57,64,65]

REFERENCES

1. Josselyn IM. The history of the American Academy of Child Psychiatry. J Am Acad Child Psychiatry 1962;1(1):196–202.
2. Ackerman NW, Sobel R. Family diagnosis: an approach to the preschool child. Am J Orthopsychiatry 1950;20(4):744–53.
3. Committee on the Family. The field of family therapy. New York: Group for the Advancement of Psychiatry; 1970.
4. Kramer DA, McKinney WT. The overlapping territories of psychiatry and ethology. J Nerv Ment Dis 1979;167(1):3–22.
5. Kramer DA, William T, McKinney J. Ethology: the natural model. Behav Brain Sci 1979;2:639–40.
6. Kramer DA. Commentary: gene-environment interplay in the context of genetics, epigenetics, and gene expression. J Am Acad Child Adolesc Psychiatry 2005; 44(1):19–27.

7. Kramer DA. Comprehensive biological treatment, i.e., CBT. AACAP News 2008; 39(1):16–7.
8. Truitt RP. The role of the child guidance clinic in the mental hygiene movement. Am J Public Health 1926;16(1):22–4.
9. Beers CW. A mind that found itself: an autobiography. New York: Longmans, Green; 1907.
10. Haynes FE. The individual delinquent. J Crim Law Criminol 1927;18(1):65–74.
11. Levy DM. Beginnings of the child guidance movement. Am J Orthopsychiatry 1968;38(5):799–804.
12. Healy W. The individual delinquent. Boston: Little, Brown, and Company; 1915.
13. Richmond JB. The pediatrician and the individual delinquent. Pediatrics 1960; 26(1):126–31.
14. Bateson G. Information and codification: a philosophical approach. In: Ruesch J, Bateson G, editors. Communication: the social matrix of psychiatry. New York: W. W. Norton & Company; 1951. p. 168–211.
15. Deutsch A. The story of GAP. New York: Group for the Advancement of Psychiatry; 1959.
16. Leopold AA. Sand County almanac. New York: Oxford University Press; 1949.
17. Tinbergen N. The study of instinct. London: Oxford University Press; 1951.
18. Ruesch J, Bateson G. Communication: the social matrix of psychiatry. New York: WW Norton; 1951.
19. Bowlby J, Robertson J. A two-year old goes to hospital. Proc R Soc Med 1953; 46(6):425–7.
20. Whitaker CA, Malone TP. The roots of psychotherapy. New York: Blakiston; 1953.
21. Kramer DA. Like (grand-) father, like (grand-) son: the implications of the transference relationship and developmentally sensitive periods for learning on the three-generational system. Denison Journal Biological Science 1988;25(1):18–35.
22. Keith DV, Kaye DL. Consultation with the extended family: Primary process in clinical practice. Child Adolesc Psychiatr Clin N Am 2001;10(3):563–76.
23. Westman JC, Cline DW, Swift WJ, et al. Role of child psychiatry in divorce. Arch Gen Psychiatry 1970;23(11):416–20.
24. Napier AY, Whitaker C. Problems of the beginning family therapist. Seminars in Psychiatry 1973;5(2):229–41.
25. Kramer DA, Anderson RB, Westman JC. The corrective autistic experience: an application of the models of Tinbergen and Mahler. Child Psychiatry Hum Dev 1984;15(2):104–20.
26. Hailman JP. How an instinct is learned. Scientific American. 1969;221(6):98–106.
27. Ackerman NW. Selected problems in supervised analysis. Psychiatry 1953;16(3): 283–90.
28. Ackerman NW. The growing edge of family therapy. In: Sager CJ, Kaplan HS, editors. Progress in group and family therapy. New York: Brunner/Mazel; 1972. p. 440–56.
29. Ackerman NW. Interpersonal disturbances in the family; some unsolved problems in psychotherapy. Psychiatry 1954;17(4):359–68.
30. Whitaker CA. Ormsby village; an experiment with forced psychotherapy in the rehabilitation of the delinquent adolescent. Psychiatry 1946;9:239–50.
31. Whitaker C. Midnight musings of a family therapist. New York: WW Norton; 1989.
32. Warkentin J, Johnson NL, Whitaker CA. A comparison of individual and multiple psychotherapy. Psychiatry 1951;14(4):415–8.
33. Lipset D. Gregory Bateson: the legacy of a scientist. Englewood Cliffs (NJ): Prentice-Hall; 1980.

34. Bateson G. Steps to an ecology of mind. New York: Ballantine; 1972.

35. Bateson G. Mind and nature: a necessary unity. New York: EP Dutton; 1979.

36. Ruesch J, Bateson G. Communication: the social matrix of psychiatry. 2nd edition. New York: WW Norton; 1968.

37. Bateson G, Jackson DD, Haley J, et al. Toward a theory of schizophrenia. Behav Sci 1956;1(4):251–64.

38. Bateson G. Minimal requirements for a theory of schizophrenia. Arch Gen Psychiatry 1960;2:477–91.

39. Bateson G. The double-bind theory–misunderstood? Psychiatr News 1978;13: 40–1.

40. Wykert J. Beyond the double bind–the schizophrenic family. Psychiatr News 1977;12:46–7.

41. Stevens JR. 'Double bind' theory. Psychiatr News 1977;12(2):11.

42. Jackson DD. The question of family homeostasis. Psychiatr Q Suppl 1957; 31(Suppl 1):79–90.

43. Wynne LC, Ryckoff IM, Day J, et al. Pseudo-mutuality in the family relations of schizophrenics. Psychiatry 1958;21(2):205–20.

44. Haley J. The family of the schizophrenic: a model system. J Nerv Ment Dis 1959; 129:357–74.

45. Jackson DD, Riskin J, Satir V. A method of analysis of a family interview. Arch Gen Psychiatry 1961;5:321–39.

46. Boszormenyi-Nagy I, Framo JL. Family concept of hospital treatment of schizophrenia. Curr Psychiatr Ther 1962;2:159–66.

47. Minuchin S, Auerswald E, King CH, et al. The study and treatment of families that produce multiple acting-out boys. Am J Orthopsychiatry 1964;34:125–33.

48. Bowen M. The use of family theory in clinical practice. Compr Psychiatry 1966; 7(5):345–74.

49. Bowlby J. Attachment and loss: volume I. Attachment. New York: Basic Books; 1969.

50. Schowalter JE. Child and adolescent psychiatry comes of age, 1944–1994. In: Menninger RW, Nemiah JC, editors. American psychiatry after World War II: (1944–1994). Washington, DC: American Psychiatric Press; 2000. p. 461–80.

51. McDermott JF Jr. Certification of the child psychiatrist. What is special about the specialist? J Am Acad Child Psychiatry 1975;14(2):196–203.

52. Gardner GE. Clinical research in a child psychiatry setting. Am J Orthopsychiatry 1956;26(2):330–9.

53. McDermott JF Jr, Char WF. The undeclared war between child and family therapy. J Am Acad Child Psychiatry 1974;13(3):422–36.

54. Keith DV, Westman JC, Whitaker CA. Contrasting child psychiatry and family therapy. Child Psychiatry Hum Dev 1988;19(2):87–97.

55. Josephson AM. Family intervention as a developmental psychodynamic therapy. Child Adolesc Psychiatr Clin North Am 2013;22(2):241–60.

56. Freeman WJ. Nonlinear brain dynamics and intention according to Aquinas. Mind Matter 2008;6(2):207–34.

57. Freeman WJ. Societies of brains: a study in the neuroscience of love and hate. Hillsdale (NJ): Lawrence Erlbaum; 1995. p. 1–26.

58. Murdock GP. Social structure. New York: Macmillan; 1949.

59. Cheney DL, Seyfarth RM. How monkeys see the world: inside the mind of another species. Chicago: The University of Chicago Press; 1990.

60. Gardner R. The social brain. Psychiatr Ann 2005;35(10):778–86.

61. Gintis H. The distributed brain. Nature 2014;509:284–5.

62. Kramer DA. The biology of family psychotherapy. Child Adolesc Psychiatr Clin North Am 2001;10(3):625–40.
63. Kramer DA. The biology of family culture. In: Combrinck-Graham L, editor. Children in family contexts. 2nd edition. New York: Guilford; 2006. p. 90–112.
64. Kramer DA. The decline of the biopsychosocial model and the demise of psychiatry. AACAP News 2012;43(3):120–1.
65. Kramer DA. DSM-5, NIMH, and the dark cave of reductionism in twenty-first century psychiatry. AACAP News 2014;45(1):18–9.
66. Bowlby J. Developmental psychiatry comes of age. Am J Psychiatry 1988;145(1): 1–10.
67. Freeman WJ. The physiology of perception. Sci Am 1991;264(2):78–85.
68. Freeman WJ. Neurodynamic models of brain in psychiatry. Neuropsychopharmacology 2003;28(Supplement 1):S54–63.
69. Asano T, Freeman WJ. How brains make up their minds: a precis in historical perspective. Mind Matter 2012;9(2):171–84.
70. Caspi A, McClay J, Moffitt TE, et al. Role of genotype in the cycle of violence in maltreated children. Science 2002;297:851–4.
71. Caspi A, Sugden K, Moffitt TE, et al. Influence of life stress on depression: moderation by a polymorphism in the 5-HTT gene. Science 2003;301:386–9.
72. Suomi SJ. How gene-environment interactions can influence emotional development in rhesus monkeys. In: Garcia-Coll C, Bearer EL, Lerner RM, editors. Nature and nurture: the complex interplay of genetic and environmental influences on human behavior and development in rhesus monkeys. Mahwah (NJ): Lawrence Erlbaum; 2004. p. 35–51.
73. Tienari P, Wynne LC, Laksy K, et al. Genetic boundaries of the schizophrenia spectrum: evidence from the Finnish Adoptive Family Study of Schizophrenia. Am J Psychiatry 2003;160(9):1587–94.
74. Tienari P, Wynne LC, Sorri A, et al. Genotype-environment interaction in schizophrenia-spectrum disorder. Long-term follow-up study of Finnish adoptees. Br J Psychiatry 2004;184:216–22.
75. Weaver IC, Cervoni N, Champagne FA, et al. Epigenetic programming by maternal behavior. Nat Neurosci 2004;7(8):847–54.
76. Buchen L. In their nurture. Nature 2010;467(7312):146–8.

From Family Therapy to Family Intervention

Allan M. Josephson, MD

KEYWORDS

- Family therapy • Family intervention • Developmental psychopathology

KEY POINTS

- Clinical work with the family must always be part of the identity of the child and adolescent psychiatrist.
- In every case, the child psychiatrist should evaluate for family vulnerabilities and coexisting family strengths.
- The family regulates affect and behavior and shapes the formation of mind.
- The child psychiatrist should assess and intervene with the family enough to understand the patient's context, to communicate with nonmedical colleagues, and to avoid diagnostic errors.
- Families are a core component of resilience: they confer genetic/experiential protection against genetic/experiential risk.

The term, *family therapy*, has been part of psychiatric lexicon for several generations, yet it may have outlived its usefulness. For many, the term conjures up the notion of all family members being present for each session, but the field has been moving away from this very specific meaning. The seminal idea of the "family as a system" is no longer the sole theory guiding family work. The systemic perspective sees individuals in a family system as interdependent, with no change occurring in a family without everything else changing accordingly. Analogous to the overreach of interpretation in the history of psychoanalysis, systems interpretations became overused.

Although the system remains a viable and important construct, there are now other ways that clinicians work with families. Some of the terms used to encompass this trend include *family treatment, family-centered treatment, relational processes and disorders, family psychiatry, family skills enhancement, family intervention science,* and *parent management training.*[1]

The term family therapy has become problematic in that, for some, it communicates that it is the province of the nonmedical therapist, marginalizing its significance.

No disclosures.
Bingham Clinic, Division of Child and Adolescent Psychiatry, Department of Pediatrics, University of Louisville School of Medicine, 200 East Chestnut Street, Louisville, KY 40202, USA
E-mail address: Allan.josephson@louisville.edu

Child Adolesc Psychiatric Clin N Am 24 (2015) 457–470
http://dx.doi.org/10.1016/j.chc.2015.02.002
1056-4993/15/$ – see front matter © 2015 Elsevier Inc. All rights reserved.
childpsych.theclinics.com

Ironically, the family's systemic properties are congruent with numerous physiologic mechanisms (eg, increase of heart rate with a drop in blood pressure). Equally problematic, for many clinicians, family therapy communicates a specialized set of skills, even esoteric, that many practitioners feel ill equipped to implement. This article proposes the use of the term, *family intervention*, to encompass the many ways contemporary clinicians work with families beyond the activities connoted by family therapy.

Family intervention is defined as a coordinated set of clinical practices designed to alter family interaction, family environment, and parental executive function. This collaborative intervention utilizes parents, child, and siblings to strengthen protective factors and mitigate family risk factors associated with child and adolescent psychiatric disorders. In addition to the amelioration of symptoms, family interventions typically address any factor that impedes child and adolescent development.

Contemporary clinicians face a question not contemplated in previous generations: what is a family? There are many changes in the contemporary family that are fully reviewed by Sargent.[2] For the purposes of this article, the term, *family*, refers to individuals who have regular contact with its children and assume the responsibility of meeting their developmental and emotional needs. The term family implies biological, affective, and legal bonds, occurring together or separately. The term, *parent*, refers to the individuals who make decisions on behalf of children. In this article, the terms, *child* and *children*, refer to any individual younger than 18 years of age; hence, the use of child includes adolescents.

The family must be considered in each case. Avoiding family work, under the guise, "I don't do family therapy," is not an option. In each clinical encounter, the clinician must consider the ways in which the family ameliorates or exacerbates psychiatric symptoms. What is the most appropriate family intervention? What are the target points for a family intervention? Who implements it? What is the knowledge base required of a clinician for a safe and effective intervention? This article responds to these questions and prepares readers for this issue's discussion of family work in specific disorders by providing an overview of the next paradigm in family treatment.

CHALLENGES FOR THE CLINICIAN MAKING A FAMILY INTERVENTION

Many contemporary challenges take psychiatric clinicians away from a family focus. These include but are not limited to

- The promise and peril of empiricism. "Not everything that counts can be counted, and not everything that can be counted, counts" (Einstein).[3]
- Family-based treatments must follow the available evidence, yet there are helpful family interventions that may not have been studied. Such interventions, addressing known risk factors, cannot be assumed to lack efficacy.
- The frequent use of medications, and the aggressive marketing of them,[4] has directed attention away from psychosocial interventions.[5,6]
- Reductionism limits seeing the big picture.[7–11] Scull has noted, "a simplistic biological reductionism has increasingly ruled the psychiatric roost. Patients and their families learned to attribute mental illness to faulty biochemistry…It was biobabble as deeply misleading and unscientific as the psychobabble it replaced."[12]
- Contemporary psychiatry provides less time for understanding patients, gathering developmental histories, and carefully developing clinical case formulations.
- The "med check" approach severely limits a gathering of data that allows a family formulation.
- Psychiatric diagnoses often lack relational context and suffer from oversimplification. Disorders are reified when a developmental explanation is more

appropriate.[13] If the symptoms of dysregulated children were seen as a regulation failure instead of a major mental illness, the bipolar epidemic could have been avoided.[14,15]

- The excitement of neuroscience discoveries is a legitimate factor decreasing emphasis on all psychosocial factors, including the family.[16]

THE FAMILY AS AN INTEGRATING PRINCIPLE OF DEVELOPMENT

Family factors must be integrated into all treatment plans. Clarification between eclecticism and integration is in order. Eclecticism is a pragmatic approach to a case in which the ingredients of different approaches are used without concern for theory. If it works, try it. On the other hand, integration assumes a more extensive blending of approaches into a broader theory.[17,18] This article describes a family approach that integrates diverse aspects of development and developmental psychopathology into a systems/developmental view of the family. It takes a broader view than a recent article that delineated a specific integration between psychodynamic, developmental, and family concepts.[19]

In child and adolescent clinical work, development must be central to any integration theory. Child psychiatry has moved from a focus on psychoanalysis in the first half of the past century to a shift to the child in the system in the latter half of the century.[20,21] Both these approaches consider development as important. The field's contemporary challenge is to integrate the facts of the clinical history, including assessment scales and rating scales, yet not lose the narrative/story of the child in family context. Carlson and Meyer[22] illustrated this challenge when they noted, "the diagnosis of bipolar disorder is often made by mindlessly applying criteria without understanding developmental history and context."

So what is developmental psychopathology? There are numerous definitions but all include the process of a child facing developmental tasks requiring mastery and a range of risk factors that impede development and a range of protective factors that foster it.[23,24] The organism/child is in interaction with the environment. Treatment efforts then are rationally directed toward decreasing environmental stress and increasing organism resilience (eg, moving a child to a less demanding classroom, increasing attentional processes through medication, and learning coping strategies). The concept of resilience—"the capacity of a dynamic system to adapt successfully to disturbances that threaten system function, viability, or development"[25(p10)]—merges with the concept of developmental psychopathology.[26]

It is widely accepted that genetically programmed developmental tasks unfold without interruption. As Masten has commented, "societies and families have observed over generations that these developmental milestones signify that a child is on track to do okay in the future. There is popular belief that competence begets competence in these developmental tasks."[25(p19)] Here is the family integrating principle again: children do not develop in vitro but in vivo. They develop in the context of the family, and family processes can dramatically foster this development or significantly impinge on it. In the former, the family operates as a protective factor and in the latter a risk factor. These developmental tasks are sequential and cumulative. Success in one area of development begets success in the next.

In behavioral studies of resilience, successful outcomes are defined as competence in age-salient developmental tasks.[25(p16)] There is general acceptance of the following common age-related, chronologic developmental tasks. Although acknowledgment goes to Erik Erikson,[27] numerous developmentalists have subsequently elaborated on his ideas.[28]

1. Infancy: establishing a social bond, a sense of basic trust, and security
2. Establishing a sense of autonomy, early independence, and self-control of impulses
3. Developing socialization, enculturation, and early peer relationships
4. Establishing a sense of productivity and achievement through burgeoning physical and intellectual skills
5. Adjusting to physical maturation; forming close, emerging romantic relationships; and independence from family

In sum, a family intervention must facilitate task mastery by mobilizing family strengths (protective factors) and by mitigating family weaknesses/problems (risk factors). Any intervention that achieves this effect inevitably ameliorates clinical symptoms.

PREPARING FOR INTERVENTION
Family Assessment

The data on which a family formulation is based are derived from a comprehensive assessment of family structure, family communication, family regulation of child development, individual functioning of child and parent, marital functioning, and the stages of the family life cycle. The data are best gathered by thorough history taking and observation of family interaction.[29,30]

The simultaneous gathering of the facts of a clinical history and observing family interaction is difficult for many clinicians. The number of individuals involved in a family interview can seem overwhelming. Ironically, the assessment process can be simplified, and even efficient, by observing family interactions play out in a consulting room. Apparent complexity can dissolve with such observations as the parent of an oppositional child asking a child's permission to comply, an overinvolved parent speaking regarding an adolescent's health concerns (eg, "Dr, we are having trouble with our periods."), or an enraged, entitled adolescent cursing at a parent.

The Practice Parameter for the Assessment of the Family (American Academy of Child and Adolescent Psychiatry) offers a helpful structured guide to eliciting a family history.[31] Other sources also describe family assessment in detail.[32,33] For disorders seen as primarily biological (eg, autism) in origin, families are seen as stressed and responding to the disorder. In other disorders with strong psychosocial underpinnings (eg, conduct disorder), the nature of family interactional sequences and parenting practices seemed to give rise to disorder.[34] In individual cases, there is often a key sequence of interactional events that culminate in the need for clinical intervention. When the assessments of individual parents, marital functioning, and the family as a unit are conducted as part of an evaluation of a child's disorder, the gathered data are always directed toward understanding and treating the child's problems.

Although some family assessments may be abbreviated (eg, straightforward attentional disorder), it is imperative in certain situations to conduct a full exploration of family functioning. These include instances in which assessment reveals:

- History of significant parental risk factors (eg, parental substance abuse or marital discord)
- History of specific family interactional problems (eg, intrafamilial aggression or child oppositional behavior)
- Observations of problematic parent-child interactions (eg, harsh parental limit setting or an overly close parent-child relationship)
- Minimal progress in an individual psychotherapeutic treatment or a pharmacologic treatment. This indication for in-depth family assessment seems more

prominent in contemporary psychiatry due to the challenges of contemporary psychiatry discussed previously.

- Another family member with psychiatric symptoms

The Practice Parameter also provides a guide to observing basic elements of family functioning.[31(p932–34)] Family structure refers to hierarchy and power relationships and the invisible boundaries within families. Family communication refers to the clarity and directness of communication and whether the content of communication is congruent with accompanying affect. Family regulation connotes how the family regulates development, specifically affect and behavior.[29] This regulation, performed externally by the family, ultimately becomes an internal regulatory process within the child and is a crucial developmental achievement.[35] Anders has provided a categorization of the regulatory process that is particularly helpful when applied to each developmental stage.[36]

Formulation

The clinical case formulation is essential for effective family intervention. It is a tool for child and adolescent psychiatrists to determine how families protect and how they pose risk for the emergence of a mental disorder. The effective formulation goes beyond a mere listing of facts and maps out how an organism/child interacts with the environment through consideration of specific factors in each category. The clinical formulation is always consistent with available empirical evidence yet can go beyond it. Effective formulations use clinical evidence understood through the lens of developmental and systems theory. A formulation of parental overprotectiveness can rationally be based on the clinical observation of a parent answering questions for a teenage child in a family therapy session. **Table 1** summarizes the factors to be considered in developing a case formulation.

Key principles of the family-oriented case formulation:

1. There is an interactional basis (organism-environment) to child psychopathology. A learning disordered child with problems in mathematics only becomes stressed when academic challenge unmasks the disability. A dependent child in an enmeshed family only develops a full-blown depression when leaving home to attend university. Effective family interventions must consider decreasing environmental stress and increasing organism resilience.
2. The behavioral and affective processes of psychological development are regulated by families. A behaviorally disordered child is observed on an inpatient unit during a parental visit. The mother rests on the child's bed, reading a magazine, making only a mild entreaty to stop her child's disruptiveness and destructive play.
3. Family experience shapes mental function (ie, family interaction becomes part of the child's mind). As an example, a teenage girl scratches her wrist and offers the cryptic comment, "I wanted to make a friend suffer." Therapy revealed an entitlement born of an adoring, almost worshipful mother, an attitude the girl came to believe others shared.
4. A formulation suggests weighing clinical variables of importance, emphasizing those with most impact on the clinical disorder. Family factors may be crucial in a serious behavior disorder and less so in a straightforward case of attentional problems.

A family-based formulation must offer a template for understanding the family factors that predispose to, precipitate, and perpetuate clinical problems. Family interaction can predispose to problems through life experience that is internalized and becomes part of the self (eg, physical abuse leading to paranoia). Family stressors, such

Table 1
Toward developing a family-based case formulation

Current picture of individual characteristics of the child	
Biological (capacities)	1. General health status 2. Medical disorder/genetic vulnerability 3. Temperament 4. Intelligence 5. Information processing/perceptual (eg, attentional process, peripheral sensory, neuropsychological) 6. Uneven development (eg, precocious sexuality, delayed speech)

Psychological (motivations/cognitive set)	1. Mastery of age-related psychosocial tasks
	  a. Trust, quality of attachment
	  b. Autonomy, separation from others
	  c. Peers, differentiation of relationships, conscience formation, empathy toward others
	  d. Achievement, sense of competence, self-esteem formation
	  e. Identity, sexual competence
	2. Has the family regulated these tasks in a balanced manner?
	3. What ongoing family interactional experiences have predisposed the child to the mastery of develop mental tasks or impeded such mastery?
	4. What ongoing family interactional experiences have predisposed the child to develop adaptive cognitive sets or maladaptive cognitive sets?
	5. How have these maladaptive cognitive sets affected developmental task mastery?
	6. Have family factors/parent-related dynamics perpetuated problems or strengths?
	7. Have family factors affected child coping strategies?

Environmental stressors	
Social (environmental demand)	1. Family factors (acute): divorce, custody battle, family geographic moves, unemployment, and poverty 2. Interpersonal: peer difficulties 3. Educational: demands outstripping ability 4. Developmental: new expectations, traumatic experiences 5. Cultural disruption (acute): war, environmental disaster 6. Cultural expectation (chronic): pressure to conform behavior to societal norms

Adapted from Josephson AM. Family intervention as a developmental psychodynamic therapy. Child Adolesc Psychiatr Clin N Am 2013;22:249; with permission.

as violence and family moves, can acutely precipitate disorder. Finally, chronic family interactions inevitably perpetuate disorders, a long-held tenet of family systems therapy. The resistance of such fixed family patterns to therapeutic change is often fueled by the internalized world of the parents, often corresponding to relationship problems of parents.[37,38] On the other hand, family strengths can protect children from the onset and evolution of these problems.

A thorough formulation helps determine whether families are primarily in need of supportive education or encouragement of behavioral change. The disease model of contemporary psychiatry typically emphasizes psychoeducation. These principles include assisting the family in recognizing onset of illness, understanding relapse, describing the effects and side effects of medications, and supporting the family's strengths as it deals with significant mental illness. This, of course, is an approach that should not be used in a family life experience model where family members must change how they relate to another and parents must change parenting practices.[39]

The first approach educates and empathically supports a family dealing with an illness. The second approach identifies problematic interactions, explores issues, and empathically challenges a family to change its manner of relating. This polarity, an either/or statement, is for heuristic purposes only. In reality, all families have strengths and weaknesses, and clinical work often involves both support and challenge. There are specific areas of inquiry that can help clinicians decide when to explore family problems and expect change and when to educate the family and offer support.[31]

INDICATIONS FOR FAMILY TREATMENT

Although families should be involved with all psychiatric treatments, there are specific indications for a focused family intervention:

1. The clinical presentation is an interactional problem. Problems, such as physical and sexual abuse, aggression directed toward a parent, a child running away from home, an eating disorder, or separation anxiety all present as interactional problems. Given that almost any childhood behavior problem is interactional and disruptive behavior is the most common problem faced by child psychiatrists, the indications for family interventions are frequent.
2. Parental psychopathology precludes effective parenting. Many times parenting strategies are not effective due to the problems of parents, including disorders such as substance abuse, aggressive behavior, and personality psychopathology. A family focus is indicated when there is a mismatch between parental personality style and child temperament.
3. Psychiatric disorders with identified family contributions. Research in developmental psychopathology and family treatment outcome studies demonstrates that there are family concomitants of many disorders that are becoming more clearly defined.[34]
4. Psychiatric disorders requiring psychoeducation. It is recognized that disorders, such as major depression, schizophrenia, and attention deficit disorder, have strong biological loadings. Education about the disorders and guiding a family's response to their family member is an important intervention. Even though family processes are not seen as directly etiologically important in some of these illnesses, relapses have been documented to occur in the absence of family intervention.[34]

MAKING THE INTERVENTION: HOW FAMILY THERAPY WORKS[1]

The evidence of the effectiveness of family interventions is growing rapidly[40,41] and is discussed elsewhere in this issue in the article by Sharma and Sargent. In most instances, the clinical issue is not should one intervene with families but how to do so, when to do so, how to sequence the intervention with other interventions, and how to intervene for specific disorders. Family interventions can range from brief history gathering episodes, to focused parent education, to extensive individual and

---

[1] This section *Adapted from* Josephson.[19]

family explorations. In making an intervention, the clinician should ask what is impeding a child's development. For example, the work of Weissman and colleagues has demonstrated that treating maternal depression is associated with the remission of child psychopathology.[42] As a result, this intervention qualifies as a family intervention.

The following section illustrates the sequencing and coordinating aspects of a family intervention. Each of these stages does not occur in every treatment nor do they always occur in the sequence listed, but in more extensive treatments all may be required.

Address Immediate Needs

Many families come to a clinic wanting to leave with something that can be done for their child that day. The presenting problem can require urgent attention. Crises may involve environmental interventions, such as removing a child from the home, most commonly by hospitalization. Although not always indicated, pharmacotherapy is increasingly offered as an immediate intervention by many clinicians, fueled by the expectations of contemporary parents. In all nonemergent initial contacts, parents need their anxieties addressed by a treatment plan: a clear description of the nature of the child's problem, what can be done about it, a time frame for change, and the family's role in the process.

This stage may include a focused behavioral intervention for conditions such as substance abuse disorders, conduct disorders, and anxiety disorders (these topics are also discussed elsewhere in this issue by Spirito and colleagues, Zajac and colleagues, and Anderson and colleagues). A well-timed behavioral intervention, consistently applied with fidelity to a protocol, may be enough to stabilize a patient.

Parent Management Training

Parent management training, supported by a growing outcome literature,[43–45] is not traditionally seen as family therapy. Yet parents are the "executives" of the family and change must start with them. Many parents, through lack of experience or their own emotional issues, do not know fundamentals of child development. Furthermore, they often need to be informed of factors related to the onset of disorder, the course of disorder, and what the family needs to do to effectively manage it. This parent education phase is important in disorders with significant biological aspects, such as disorders of attention and learning.

Given the commonality of disruptive behavior problems, parents need a working knowledge of behavior management principles. In milder problems, education and parent management are often all that are necessary. In cases of more serious psychopathology, parental vulnerabilities often preclude the effective implementation of behavior management strategies. For example, a mother's depression and dependency often make limit setting difficult, or a father's anger and aggression may undo the effective limit setting efforts of the mother. When such events are observed, it can lead to a broadening of therapy. The clinician formulates what needs to change in the family, and empathically holds the family accountable to change, while appreciating its difficulty. Often a next step is seeing the family together.

Intervention in Family Process

Intervening in family processes most closely resembles traditional family therapy. All family members living in a household are invited to attend and the clinician guides the family in altering problematic interactions between family members. Common interventions include shoring up parental support of each other when a child is disrespectful to one parent; encouraging parents' authoritative, deliberate limit setting in lieu of a friendly, deferential response; identifying how one parent may undermine the other in limit setting efforts; and facilitating an engagement with a child when there may be evidence of a parent being unempathic to a child's distress. Empathically intervening in various family processes can have a significant impact on family and individual functioning.

For a generation, family systems therapy emphasized various techniques and described these techniques in a voluminous literature.[46,47] Interventions using techniques, such as reframing problems and circular questioning, can be particularly useful in elucidating interpersonal dynamics and the intrapsychic dynamics of specific family members. Often, however, these types of interventions are met with resistance. Systems theory suggests that family homeostasis is the desired state, yet careful study of the individuals in the family often reveals they have their own reasons for resisting change.[48] For example, in setting a limit on a child and experiencing the child's natural resistance, a parent may experience fears of being abandoned by the child. Understanding such fears may require an individual intervention with a parent. When altering family interaction is successful (eg, parents are more effective in setting limits or more engaged with their child), the internalized world of the child shaped by previous dysfunctional interactions may require individual intervention.

Individual Intervention

Change in family interaction is often resisted due to the inner world of parents, which have to be altered if family interactions are to change. By keeping parents' internal working models constant, family interactions perform a defensive, protective function for the parents. The effect of enhancing parental self efficacy through an individual intervention can be heightened when coupled with altering family relationships and parent education. It is always important for a child clinician to remember when intervening with a parent to relate the work to the needs of the identified child patient.

Successful family interaction work often unmasks a child whose inner world has been shaped by family interactions. A child's inner world stems from family interactions but, as development unfolds, has a life independent from those interactions. This inner world requires an individual psychotherapeutic intervention. For example, a child who has been persistently indulged in a family context likely has a sense of entitlement needing clinical attention.

Marital/Couple Interventions

Given that the parents' decisions set the stage for many family interactions, a marital and couple intervention flows from family interventions that are resisted or ineffective. Driven by their internal working models, parents may unwittingly continue to facilitate dysfunctional interactions between themselves, powerfully affecting their children. One parent may have a helpful parenting perspective but may be undermined by the other, only to have these roles shift in another context. Working on communication styles and parenting can be the prelude for couples to be seen alone to explore their individual perspectives on parenting and identify individual parental vulnerabilities.

Dealing with Siblings

It is not uncommon for family work, initially focused on an identified patient, to indicate that there is another child needing intervention. This child is subjected to the same family dynamics but may have responded differently due to individual variables (eg, biologic differences in attention and learning, birth order, gender, or step-sibling status). In addition to gaining attention to their own needs, siblings can often provide a unique perspective on the problems of their sibling, helping parents see things in a different light. They may not be actively involved in regular sessions; however, an initial assessment and other intermittent contacts can flesh out the clinician's understanding of the family.

In sum, the order of these interventions is flexible, and they may not all be needed in each situation. In certain situations, one therapist can sequentially provide all therapies; in others, multiple therapists need to be involved for pragmatic, if not theoretic, reasons. The issue of the number of therapists and their relationship with each other remains one of some contention but perhaps less so than in a previous generation. Readers are referred elsewhere for a more complete discussion.[49,50]

CLINICAL VIGNETTE

Case Illustration of Intervention Sequencing

Blaine was a 10-year, 10-month-old fifth-grade student seen for a second psychiatric opinion of moodiness, fears, and rages "when he doesn't get his way." At the time of psychiatric consultation, the parents—Michael and Janet—saw Blaine as not being able to control his behavior; his mother believed he was "suffering." When angry, he would slam doors, curse, and yell for periods of time, as long as 1 hour in duration. Managing his rages, related to homework expectations, was difficult and emotionally draining for the parents, because it would often take 3 hours for Blaine to complete his homework. Blaine had been in treatment for more than 1 year with little progress, and his parents were frustrated, as well as fearful, about the effects of his "bipolar disorder." Treatment consisted solely of psychopharmacology, with little therapeutic effect, and 1 major side effect, a 25-pound weight gain.

Blaine was of average intelligence and had not failed any classes. He and his sister Laura, 2 years younger, were biracial children adopted at the time of birth by white parents. The adoptive parents had been married for 32 years; mother was 53 years old and father was 55 years old.

His parents had difficulty managing his rages when homework was required. Blaine could not finish assignments unless his mother was there, and even then he would neglect her requests, at times threatening violence. She then, in exasperation, would ask his father to help, who would encourage, cajole, and then, in anger, challenge Blaine to complete his homework. When pushed in this way, Blaine would often threaten to kill himself. During the homework sessions, Blaine would frequently verbally assault his mother, calling her stupid, ugly, crazy, and a liar, including vulgar epithets.

*Therapy began with attempts to help parents **stabilize Blaine's current behavior**. This meant ensuring Blaine's safety, and that of his parents, by doing careful interviews to assess the veracity and credibility of his verbal threats to kill himself and his parents. The parents were given instruction on how to find emergency care, although they never needed to use such care. The first phase of therapy emphasized **parent management** techniques to facilitate homework completion. The parents were encouraged in their firmness, and a positive reward system was implemented to facilitate task completion.*

*The pleasant couple wanted Blaine to complete homework uneventfully and when his distress mounted, it immobilized them. Behavioral management strategies were difficult to implement because of family psychodynamic factors, which required a **family intervention** alongside a couple intervention.*

*In **couples work**, it was revealed that mother had always wanted children, but father had not. They had been married 22 years before they finally adopted. When the children were younger, Michael adored the children. Yet as they grew older, he withdrew from active family life, spending much of his time on the computer, leaving most of the parenting tasks to his wife. Father wanted to be Blaine's friend, making discipline next to impossible. He seemed influenced by his own developmental history of "little discipline, lots of play, and no schedule." The* *therapy emphasized the need for Michael to support his wife more and to expect his wife to be less active as the primary limit setter.*

*One critical incident occurred in **family work**. Blaine physically confronted his parents after they limited his activities with an electronic game. In that session, Blaine's mother tearfully pleaded for help from her husband. As if to take on her father's role, Blaine's younger sister crossed the room and hugged her crying mother. Father verbalized that his son did not seem to understand the concept of limits and wondered why Blaine expressed no concern toward his mother. As therapy progressed and mother continued to insist that she needed support, her husband Michael became mobilized and was more supportive of her. In the couples work, Janet stated, "Mike doesn't want to deal with confrontation and the stress that inevitably results from it."*

In couples work, the parents grappled with the issue of diagnosis and medication treatment. Mother stated, "We took the view that we needed to help him control things by finding the right medicine." They acknowledged that a change in therapeutic approach to de-emphasize medication was helpful. They told the therapist that "you listened to us more, and you gave us hope. Particularly, you made us stop and look at the real parenting differences between us, and how they were related to Blaine's behavior problem. You got us moving in the right direction."

In couples work, mother was able to ventilate, stating, "I'm the more parenting person. Mike is the fun parent. This made me angry, because it left me as the only person to get things done." The therapist pursued the goal of getting mother less involved, and father more involved, using improved couple communication. Janet said, "Mike doesn't like the imposition of a schedule," and the therapist was able to point out that children need schedules. Janet pointed out that "Mike doesn't deal with conflict," while the therapist pointed out that active parenting naturally involves conflict and demands solving it.

*In **individual work**, Mike was able to see the influence of his own background. "My father wasn't around when I was growing up, and I vowed that I was going to be around more. I wasn't going to make the same mistake. I think his absence affected me. I now wish I'd been closer to my father; I might have learned more." The therapist pointed out that "you corrected but you overcorrected." Mike agreed, noting, "I have wanted to be a friend to my son, and not a parent."*

The therapist challenged Michael with the question, "When children threaten to harm a kind, caring mother, what does this mean?" He responded: "It means the child is too comfortable with not enough limits." Chagrinned, Michael came to see how he had enabled his son's tyrannical, verbally abusive behavior toward his mother. He came to understand that his joking approach led Blaine to believe most of his behavioral indiscretions "weren't that big a deal."

*Finally, **sibling work** emphasized Blaine's younger sister and her developing behavior disorder. The parent's identified Laura's noncompliance and challenging of parents to be similar to Blaine's behavior but felt reassured that with their new self-knowledge of their family's, and their own, dynamics they would have solutions to her behavioral challenges (case report reprinted from Josephson, 2013).[19]*

CHALLENGES IN IMPLENTATION

For many clinicians, seeing a family raises ethical problems. The simplest of questions focuses the main challenge: "Who is the patient?" Although therapy is initially planned for the identified patient, as family interventions proceed, the concerns and problems of other members may become a focus for treatment. When a clinician empathically explores one family member's perspective, she may be seen as alienating the patient or another family member. Healthier families understand this apparent unfairness as part of the process of therapy. Families who are influenced by psychopathology are less likely to understand this type of intervention. In those cases, the clinician makes a deliberate attempt to relate to all family members and make the point that in time each person's perspective will be heard. With integrated treatment becoming more common, these concerns may be less prominent than in the past.[50]

There are elements of clinical work that may not typically be seen as a family intervention or family therapy but are crucial in developing family stability. These include helping parents negotiate community support systems, such as in-home care for developmentally disabled children, supporting parents' efforts in procuring appropriate educational services, and communicating with the legal system.[51] Coordinating family interventions with other clinical interventions (eg, pharmacotherapy) is often needed.[52]

Aspects of race, culture, gender, sexual orientation, and worldview are important in all families.[53,54] As the influence of the traditional family wanes, how patients develop their idea of family is influenced by these various factors. Special problems, such as divorce, custody, legal issues, and violence, are increasingly prominent in contemporary society.[55] These issues and others can complicate any family intervention.

SUMMARY

The power of family therapy—all members of a family meeting to understand and help one of its child members—remains. Yet the flexible application of various aspects of treatment comprises a paradigm shift to family intervention. The power is increasingly focused on specific areas of family life. Because the family regulates affect and behavior and shapes the child's mind, the family continues to be a most formative influence on a child and adolescent's life.

REFERENCES

1. Josephson AM. Reinventing family therapy: teaching family intervention as a new treatment modality. Acad Psychiatry 2008;32(5):405–13.
2. Sargent J. Variations in family composition: implications for family therapy. Child Adolesc Psychiatr Clin N Am 2001;10:577–99.
3. Einstein A. 2008. Available at: http://en.wikiquote.org/AlbertEinstein. Accessed March 19, 2015.
4. Fournier JC, DeRubeis RJ, Hollon SD, et al. Antidepressant drug effects and depression severity: a patient-level meta-analysis. JAMA 2010;202(1):47–53.
5. Spielman GI, Parry PI. From evidence-based medicine to marketing-based medicine: the evidence from internal industry documents. J Bioeth Inq 2010;7:13–29.
6. Boyce P. Restoring wisdom to the practice of psychiatry. Australas Psychiatry 2006;14:3–7.
7. Kramer DA. DSM-5, NIMH, and the dark cave of reductionism in twenty-first century psychiatry. AACAP News 2014;44:18–9.
8. Eisenberg L. Nature, niche, and nurture: the role of social experience in transforming genotype into phenotype. Acad Psychiatry 1998;22:213–22.
9. Silove D. Biologism in psychiatry. Aust N Z J Psychiatry 1990;24:461–3.
10. Eisenberg L. Mindlessness and brainlessness in psychiatry. Br J Psychiatry 1986; 148:497–508.
11. Rutter M. How the environment affects mental health. Br J Psychiatry 2005;186:4–6.
12. Scull A. A psychiatric revolution. Lancet 2010;375:1246–7.
13. McHugh PR. Striving for coherence: psychiatry's efforts over classification. JAMA 2005;293(20):2527–8.
14. American Academy of Child and Adolescent Psychiatry. Symposium 30: dysregulated but NOT bipolar: new insights into childhood problems with self- regulation.

2010. Available at: http://aacap.confex.com/aacap/2010/webprogram/Session 5573.html. Accessed March 19, 2015.

15. American Academy of Child and Adolescent Psychiatry. Clinical perspectives 29: when the diagnosis is bipolar: are there other explanations? 2010. p. 125–44. Available at: http://aacap.confex.com/aacap/2010/webprogram/Session4853. html. Accessed March 19, 2015.

16. Insel TR. Mental disorders in childhood: shifting the focus from behavioral symptoms to neurodevelopmental trajectories. JAMA 2014;311(17):1727–8.

17. Lebow J. Clinical theory and practice integrative family therapy: the integrative revolution in couple and family therapy. Fam Process 1997;36:1–17.

18. Lebow JL. Couple and family therapy: an integrative map of the territory. Washington, DC: American Psychological Association; 2014.

19. Josephson AM. Family intervention as a developmental psychodynamic therapy. Child Adolesc Psychiatr Clin N Am 2013;22:241–60.

20. Von Bertalanffy L. General system theory: foundations, development, applications. New York: George Braziller; 1968.

21. McDermott J, Char W. The undeclared war between child and family therapy. J Am Acad Child Adolesc Psychiatry 1974;13:422–36.

22. Carlson GA, Meyer SE. Phenomenology and diagnosis of bipolar disorder in children, adolescents, and adults: complexities and developmental issues. Dev Psychopathol 2006;18:939–69.

23. Kim-Cohen J. Resilience and developmental psychopathology. Child Adolesc Psychiatr Clin N Am 2007;16:271–83.

24. Kendler KS, Ohlsson H, Sundquist K, et al. Peer deviance, parental divorce, and genetic risk in the prediction of drug abuse in a nationwide Swedish sample: evidence of environment-environment and gene-environment interaction. JAMA Psychiatry 2014;7(14):439–45.

25. Masten AS. Ordinary magic: resilience in development. New York: Guilford Press; 2014.

26. Luthar S. Resilience in development: a synthesis of research across five decades. In: Cicchetti D, Cohen D, editors. Developmental psychopathology. 2nd edition. Hoboken (NJ): Wiley & Sons; 2006. p. 739–95.

27. Erikson E. Childhood and society. New York: Norton; 1963.

28. Bowlby J. A secure base: parent-child attachment and healthy human development. New York: Basic Books; 1988.

29. Josephson A, Moncher F. Observation, interview and mental status assessment (OIM): family unit and subunits. In: Noshpitz J, editor. Handbook of child and adolescent psychiatry, vols. 5, 62. New York: John Wiley and Sons; 1998. p. 393–414.

30. Josephson A, Moncher F. Family history. In: Noshpitz J, editor. Handbook of child and adolescent psychiatry, vols. 5, 48. New York: John Wiley and Sons; 1998. p. 284–96.

31. American Academy of Child and Adolescent Psychiatry Work Group on Quality Issues, Josephson AM. Practice parameter for the assessment of the family. J Am Acad Child Adolesc Psychiatry 2007;46:922–37.

32. Wendel R, Gouze KR. Family therapy: assessment and intervention. In: Dulcan MK, editor. Dulcan's textbook of child and adolescent psychiatry. Washington, DC: American Psychiatric Publishing; 2010. p. 869–86.

33. Gouze KR, Wendel R. Integrative module-based family therapy: application and training. J Marital Fam Ther 2008;34:269–86.

34. Diamond G, Josephson A. Family-based treatment research: a 10-year update. J Am Acad Child Adolesc Psychiatry 2005;44:872–87.

35. Committee on Integrating the Science of Early Childhood Development. Acquiring self-regulation. In: Shonkoff J, Phillips D, editors. From neurons to neighborhoods: the science of early childhood development. 2nd edition. Washington, DC: National Academy Press; 2001. p. 93–123.
36. Anders T. Clinical syndromes, relationship disturbances, and their assessment. In: Sameroff A, Emde R, editors. Relationship disturbances in early childhood: a developmental approach. New York: Basic Books; 1989. p. 125–44.
37. Malone C. Child and adolescent psychiatry and family therapy: an overview. Child Adolesc Psychiatr Clin N Am 2001;10:395–414.
38. Josephson A, Moncher F. Family treatment. In: Noshpitz J, editor. Handbook of child and adolescent psychiatry, vols. 6, 16. New York: John Wiley and Sons'; 1998. p. 294–312.
39. Josephson A. Working with families: toward a common sense empathy. JACAAP News 1996;28:46–7.
40. Diamond G, Serano A, Dicky M, et al. Empirical support for family therapy. J Am Acad Child Adolesc Psychiatry 1996;35:6–16.
41. Kaslow N, Robbins Broth M, Oyeshiku Smith C, et al. Family-based interventions for child and adolescent disorders. J Marital Fam Ther 2012; 38:82–100.
42. Weissman M, Pilowsky D, Wickramaratne P, et al. Remissions in maternal depression and child psychopathology. JAMA 2006;295:1389–97.
43. Kazdin A. Practitioner review: psychosocial treatments for conduct disorder in children. J Child Psychol Psychiatry 1997;38:161–78.
44. Forehand RL, McMahon RJ. Helping the noncompliant child: a clinician's guide to parent training. New York: Guilford; 1981.
45. Eyeberg SM, Boggs SR. Parent-child interaction therapy: a psychosocial intervention for the treatment of young conduct-disordered children. In: Briesmeister JM, Schaeffer CE, editors. Handbook of parent training: parents as co-therapists for children's behavior problems. New York: Wiley; 1998. p. 61–97.
46. Minuchin S, Fishman H. Family therapy techniques. Cambridge (MS): Harvard University Press; 2004.
47. Haley J, Hoffman L. Techniques of family therapy. New York: Basic Books, Inc; 1967.
48. Nichols M. The self in the system: expanding the limits of family therapy. New York: Brunner/Mazel; 1987.
49. Josephson A, Serrano A. The integration of individual therapy and family therapy in the treatment of child and adolescent psychiatric disorders. Child Adolesc Psychiatr Clin N Am 2001;10:431–50.
50. Glick I, Berman E, Clarkin J, et al. Marital and family therapy. 4th edition. Washington: American Psychiatric Press, Inc; 2000. p. 683–99.
51. Combrinck-Graham L. Children in families in communities. Child Adolesc Psychiatr Clin N Am 2001;10:613–24.
52. Sprenger D, Josephson A. Integration of pharmacotherapy and family therapy in the treatment of children and adolescents. J Am Acad Child Adolesc Psychiatry 1998;37(8):887–9.
53. Josephson A, Peteet J, editors. Handbook of spirituality and worldview in clinical practice. Washington, DC: American Psychiatric Publishing, Inc; 2004.
54. Josephson A, Dell M. Religion and spirituality in child and adolescent psychiatry: a new frontier. Child Adolesc Psychiatr Clin N Am 2004;13(1):1–15.
55. Keitner G, Heru A, Glick I. Clinical manual of couples and family therapy. Washington, DC: American Psychiatric Publishing, Inc; 2010.

Overview of the Evidence Base for Family Interventions in Child Psychiatry

Neha Sharma, DO*, John Sargent, MD

KEYWORDS

- Family therapy • Family intervention • Children • Adolescent • Mental health
- Parent training

KEY POINTS

- There is sufficient evidence to support that family involvement is effective in managing child and adolescent mental health issues.
- There is some evidence to show that family involvement in treatment results in maintenance of posttreatment improvement.
- Chronic and refractory conditions, such as conduct disorder, substance abuse, and delinquency, can be effectively treated with family therapy–based treatments, such as multisystemic therapy, functional family therapy, and multidimensional family therapy.

METHOD OF THIS REVIEW

This article reviews randomized controlled trials (RCTs) for family-based interventions carried out over the last 15 years. The studies were selected from an evidence-based clearinghouse search for family therapy, and specific child and adolescent psychiatric disorders. Thus, it is a selective review guided by exposure to as many well done RCTs as possible that evaluate major schools of family intervention and/or different types of family therapy. Family interventions can be quite variable in their level of intensity; therefore, this article is organized from least intensive to most intensive treatment.

INTRODUCTION

The development of family therapy began in the years following World War II. Although experts in family therapy found it to be an effective treatment of mental health issues especially for children and adolescents, it was consistently criticized for a lack of

The authors have nothing to disclose.
Department of Psychiatry, Tufts Medical Center, 800 Washington Street, Boston, MA 02111, USA
* Corresponding author. 800 Washington Street, #1007, Boston, MA 02111.
E-mail address: nsharma@tuftsmedicalcenter.org

Child Adolesc Psychiatric Clin N Am 24 (2015) 471–485
http://dx.doi.org/10.1016/j.chc.2015.02.011
1056-4993/15/$ – see front matter © 2015 Elsevier Inc. All rights reserved.

childpsych.theclinics.com

Abbreviations	
ABFT	Attachment-based family therapy
ADHD	Attention-deficit/hyperactivity disorder
AFT	Adolescent-focused individual therapy
AGT	Adolescent group therapy
ASD	Autism spectrum disorder
CBT	Cognitive behavioral therapy
CCT	Client-centered therapy
FBT	Family-based treatment
FCBT	Family cognitive behavioral treatment
FESA	Family-based education, support, and attention
FFT	Functional family therapy
FPE	Family psychoeducation
ICBT	Individual cognitive behavior treatment
MDFT	Multidimensional family therapy
MEI	Multifamily educational intervention
MST	Multisystemic therapy
MTFC	Multidimensional treatment foster care
PTSD	Posttraumatic stress disorder
RAP-P	Resourceful adolescent parent program
RCTs	Randomized controlled trials
TF-CBT	Trauma-focused cognitive behavioral therapy

empirical data demonstrating its efficacy. However, over the last two decades, research in the effectiveness of family therapy and family interventions has been steadily increasing.

COMMON FACTORS

All family interventions possess some common features, such as a willingness to connect with the family and to develop a shared vision of family success in solving the problem. Successful engagement with the family not only requires dedicated professionals with a shared vision, treatment plan, and constant monitoring, but also an interest in and understanding of the family's strengths and limitations. The family and the clinician form a team that facilitates parental collaboration and agrees on roles of each individual in the treatment with the aim to empower families toward self-care and self-direction. This change requires a deep and intense engagement by the therapist resulting in new patterns for the family.

To create new and more adaptive patterns, the therapist must strive to forge a systemic therapeutic alliance with the families. The focus is to develop parenting, cognitive, behavioral, and problem-solving skills in the participants such that the presenting symptoms decline and the newly learned skills are reinforced by the parents. The aim is to enhance positive interactions by improving communication skills, building connections, identifying strengths, sharing emotions, developing shared concerns, maintaining focus, and increasing willingness to be direct. The therapist helps families to develop conflict resolution skills, and the skills to manage affect among family members. Overall, the goal is that family members learn to build positive attachment and connections so that they can provide mutual support for each other while also connecting with community support, services, and systems.

Different mental health challenges among children and adolescents require specific responses from parents, caretakers, and family members to improve. Anxiety requires parental confidence and security. Depression requires parental attachment and availability. Disruptive disorders require parental authority, supervision, and consistency. Trauma-related problems require parents to provide safety and see the problem through the eyes of the child. Eating disorders require parental collaboration and consistency. Autism spectrum disorders (ASDs) require parental understanding, acceptance, and the capacity to collaborate with other involved professionals. These realities provide a direction for family interventions and are at the heart of evidence-based treatments.

SOME APPROACHES TO SPECIFIC PROBLEMS WITH RANDOMIZED CONTROLLED TRIAL EVIDENCE

The different approaches are organized from least intensive to most intensive.

Family Psychoeducation for Adolescent Depression

How family psychoeducation (FPE) impacts different child and adolescent mental health issues varies depending on the condition. Sanford and colleagues[1] attempted to answer this question specifically for adolescent depression through an unblinded RCT. They assessed the outcome of FPE for acute depressive symptoms in the adolescent and the improvement in family and social functioning by studying two groups. Both groups received the "usual treatment," which can include individual counseling, group counseling, supportive case management, or drug therapy. The drug therapy was antidepressants, selective serotonin reuptake inhibitors, venlafaxine, or bupropion, in combination with anxiolytics or antipsychotics, as indicated by the case. Although both groups received different combinations of this treatment, one group was provided with 12 FPE sessions lasting 90 minutes in their home. FPE sessions included several topics, such as the medical model of understanding depression, patient education, stress vulnerability, communication, and coping models.

The power of this study is small with 16 families in the experimental group and 15 families in the control group. All adolescents had a high rate of comorbidities, such as generalized anxiety disorder, social phobia, and substance abuse. The participants had moderate to severe depression confirmed by low Children's Global Assessment Scale scores. At the posttreatment assessment, 21% of the FPE group and 50% of the control group met major depressive disorder criteria. At follow-up, these numbers increased to 25% and 53% for the FPE and control group, respectively. Improvements were noted in adolescent–mother, adolescent–father, and peer relationships. Also, parents reported improved social functioning of the adolescent. The FPE group had decrease in depressive symptoms acutely and at 3-month follow-up. It also had a better quality of relationships with parents and peers.

Parent Training for Autism Spectrum Disorder

Children with ASD struggle in social emotional development because of their inability to read and understand social cues. Because of limited language development, they often use behaviors to communicate. These behaviors can be used to express frustrations or to resist demands that are challenging. Often, parents struggle to understand these behaviors and may react to a child in a manner that reinforces the maladaptive behavior. Also, if parents do not address the behavior appropriately, they may fail to support the child in learning more adaptive skills.

There are RCTs that have looked at outcome of parent training plus medication for children with ASD. Aman and colleagues[2] found that subjects in the risperidone plus parent training group had significantly lower scores on standardized rating scale for behavior problems. Handen and colleagues[3] attempted to expand on that study by adding an observational component to better assess the improvement in behavior. They conducted a 24-week RCT of risperidone and risperidone plus parent training (COMB group). All the subjects (N = 124) had diagnosis of ASD, were of age 4 to 13, had IQ greater than or equal to 35 and mental age greater than or equal to 18 months, and had a raw score of greater than 18 on the parent-rated Aberrant Behavior Checklist for Irritability. The dose of risperidone was adjusted according to weight. If risperidone was found to be ineffective or intolerable, subjects were switched to aripiprazole. The COMB group (N = 75) received parent training from a trained behaviorist for 60 to 90 minutes weekly for 16 weeks. Three of those sessions were optional. The sessions were individualized to target the symptoms of each child, and thus each family received individualized homework. Parents also received booster face-to-face sessions and a telephone call between 16 and 24 weeks. The training emphasized preventing antecedent factors, using positive reinforcement, and teaching new skills.

The authors used the Standardized Observation Analogue Procedure to assess the outcome. The raters watched the family interact through a one-way observation room and communicated to the parent via a "bug in the ear" device. Parent–child interaction was observed at baseline and Week 24 in four conditions: (1) free play condition, (2) social attention condition, (3) demand condition, and (4) tangible restriction condition. At each condition, the child had increasingly less attention from the parent and more demand placed on them. After 24 weeks, the COMB group had the lowest rate of inappropriate behavior in the free play condition and highest rate of compliance in the demand condition. Additionally, there was increased positive reinforcement by parents during the free play and demand conditions. Parents also made significantly less restrictive statements during the social attention condition. The addition of parent training to medication management improved child's behavior and parents' supportive reactions.

Attachment-Based Treatment of Adolescent Depression

Family factors, such as a weak attachment, high hostility, parental psychopathology, and poor parenting, have been implicated in adolescent depression.[4,5] Attachment-based family therapy (ABFT) was developed by Diamond and Siqueland[6] to address these factors in treating adolescent depression. ABFT integrates elements of structural family therapy, multidimensional family therapy (MDFT), contextual therapy, emotion-focused therapy, and attachment therapy.[7] The principle of ABFT is that a negative family environment prevents adolescents from developing appropriate coping skills that would allow them to buffer social stressors. Without these coping skills, they are at risk of developing or exacerbating depressive symptoms.[8,9]

The ABFT manual that was developed for this study aligned with the goal of repairing attachment between parent and adolescent and promoting individuation. They hoped to reach that goal by following the tasks listed in **Table 1**.

To assess the effectiveness of ABFT on adolescent depression, Diamond and Siqueland[6] randomized 32 depressed participants aged between 13 and 17 years to two groups: ABFT and waitlist control for 12 weeks. Seventy-eight percent of the participants were female and were predominately African-American. Treatment was delivered by therapists who received training and weekly supervision with the first author.[10]

The participants in the ABFT group had a decrease in the diagnosis of depression and in the severity of depressive and anxious symptoms after 12 weeks of treatment.

Table 1
Attachment-based family therapy goals

Task	Problem Addressed	Goal
Relational reframe	Parent criticism	Cognitive shift from "fixing" to "improving" family relations
Adolescent alliance building	Low engagement of the adolescent	Bonding, identifying goals, and preparing adolescent to communicate with parents
Parent alliance building	Parental stress	Bonding, empathizing, and encouraging parents to be receptive to adolescent
Attachment	Past failed attachments	Rebuilding trust by listening to adolescent's anger and offering remorse
Competence-promoting	Negative self-concept	Encouragement to establish successful relationships outside of home

Adapted from Diamond GS, Reis BF, Diamond GM, et al. Attachment-based family therapy for depressed adolescents: a treatment development study. J Am Acad Child Adolesc Psychiatry 2002;41:1190–96; with permission.

The same participants reported a decrease in hopelessness and suicidal ideation. They also described improved attachment to their mother. Similarly, another study showed effectiveness of ABFT for adolescents with suicidal ideation and depression.[11]

Family-Based Cognitive Behavioral Treatment of Anxiety Disorders

There are sufficient data demonstrating that the presence of parental anxiety indicates poorer prognosis or response to treatment of the child with anxiety disorder.[12–14] Kendall and colleagues[15] hypothesized that individual cognitive behavioral treatment (ICBT) and family cognitive behavioral treatment (FCBT) would show significant improvement in comparison with family-based education, support, and attention (FESA). They also sought to answer the following questions: whether the treatment causes change in parental anxiety; and whether the presence of parental anxiety moderated child outcomes. A total of 161 subjects age 7 to 14 with diagnosis of anxiety disorder (separation anxiety disorder, generalized anxiety disorder, and social phobia) were included in this study. Therapists for each treatment group reviewed the manuals and attended two 3-hour workshops. During the study, the therapists participated in weekly 2-hour group supervision.

Each of the three treatment modalities (ICBT, FCBT, and FESA) followed manuals. Each treatment had 16 weekly 60-minute sessions. ICBT and FCBT both used Coping CAT Workbook,[16] which emphasized the FEAR acronym (F- feeling frightened; E- expecting bad things to happen; A- Attitudes and actions; R- Rewards and results), behavioral strategies, relaxation training, contingent reinforcement, and homework tasks. Both included parents in Sessions 4 and 9. However, in FCBT, the family CBT for anxious children manual was also used. This resulted in sessions that focused on modifying maladaptive parental beliefs. It included teaching parents strategies to respond to their children's anxiety in a constructive and supportive manner. This was to be done while encouraging effective communication between parents and children. In FCBT, parents and children met separately during Sessions 4 and 9 to provide an opportunity to discuss private questions. FESA relied on psychoeducation about emotions in general and theories of presentation of anxiety, and provided a setting to discuss the child's anxiety. The participants in the FESA group were not given directions on how to manage anxiety. Similar to FCBT, Sessions 4 and 9 were reserved for parents to discuss their concerns with the therapist privately.

Kendall and colleagues[15] concluded that both ICBT and FCBT were superior to FESA. This also indicates that FCBT may not be superior to ICBT; however, it is possible that inclusion of the family may have resulted in a decreased number of individual sessions required. Because parents were aware of the type of treatment their child was receiving and teachers were not, the authors chose to use teacher reports to assess reduction in symptoms. According to teacher reports, the ICBT posttreatment improvement in the child's anxiety was significantly greater than in the FCBT and FESA conditions as shown in **Fig. 1**. A 40% improvement in parental anxiety was noted, but it was not significantly different among the three treatments.

Trauma-Focused Cognitive Behavioral Therapy for Sexual Trauma

Trauma-focused cognitive behavioral therapy (TF-CBT) is a manualized treatment that contextualizes traumatic experiences for the child and the parent while teaching coping skills.[17,18] It consists of different phases that integrate gradual exposure and parental involvement throughout treatment. The first phase is a stabilization phase that includes the following components: psychoeducation, parenting skills, relaxation skills, affect regulation skills, and cognitive processing skills. The second phase is the trauma narrative development phase during which the traumatic experience is processed. The third phase is called the consolidation phase, in which there is in vivo exposure, increased parent and child conjoint sessions, and emphasis on enhancing safety. A complete discussion of TF-CBT is provided by Cohen and Mannarino.

Deblinger and colleagues[19] conducted an RCT to assess the efficacy of 12 sessions of TF-CBT compared with 12 sessions of client-centered therapy (CCT) for sexually abused 8 to 14 year olds. In this study, TF-CBT was conducted as described

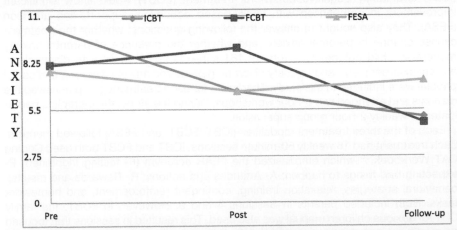

Fig. 1. Teacher's report of children's anxiety. (*From* Kendall PC, Hudson JL, Gosch E, et al. Cognitive-behavioral therapy for anxiety disordered youth: a randomized clinical trial evaluating child and family modalities. J Consulting Clinic Psychol 2008;76(2):293; with permission.)

previously. The focus of CCT was to establish a trusting relationship that enhanced self-affirmation, empowerment, and validation for both parent and child. The results of the study showed that subjects in TF-CBT (N = 92) had a significant reduction in posttraumatic stress disorder (PTSD) symptoms in comparison with subjects in CCT (N = 91). Parents reported a significant decrease in their child's behavioral problems and felt more confident about their parenting. In comparison with the CCT group, at 6- and 12-month follow-up, children and parents in the TF-CBT group maintained their gains. Additionally, there is further evidence of the efficacy of TF-CBT in 3 to 17 year olds who experienced symptoms of PTSD.[20,21] It was noted to lead to significant improvement in PTSD, depression, anxiety, cognitive, and behavior problems.[22,23]

Family-Based Treatment of Anorexia Nervosa

Lock and colleagues[24] compared manualized family-based treatment (FBT) for anorexia nervosa with adolescent-focused individual therapy (AFT). One hundred and twenty-one participants with anorexia nervosa, diagnosed by Diagnostic Standard Manual-IV criteria, aged 12 through 18 years old, were randomized to either treatment. It was not mandatory for the participants to have amenorrhea, a slight modification from Diagnostic Standard Manual-IV criteria. Both groups received 24 hours of the respective treatment over 12 months. They were assessed at baseline, end of treatment, and 6- and 12-month follow-up (discussed in more detail elsewhere in this issue). The authors concluded that significantly more participants achieved full remission (>95% ideal body weight) at 6- and 12-month follow-up in the FBT group. At the end of the treatment, participants in the FBT group reached partial remission more than AFT group. Weight gain was noted to appear faster with fewer hospitalizations for the FBT group at follow-up.

Family-Focused Treatment of Bipolar Disorder

Miklowitz and colleagues[10] conducted a study to assess whether family-focused treatment of adolescents with bipolar I or II disorders reduces the time spent ill and increases the time in remission during the year after the treatment. This study compared family-focused treatment with enhanced care while both groups received pharmacologic treatment concurrently. The pharmacologic treatment was based on standardized algorithm that reflected an up-to-date literature review. Medications were managed by board-certified psychiatrists who received monthly supervision from expert pharmacologists.

The families in the family-focused treatment group received 21 family sessions of 50 minutes. For the first 3 months, these sessions occurred weekly, then every 2 weeks for the following 3 months. Thereafter, three sessions took place every 3 months. During these sessions, families were provided with psychoeducation, communication enhancement training, and problem-solving skills training, in that order. In comparison, participants in the enhanced care arm received an abbreviated version of the family-focused treatment manual with a focus on moods and relapse prevention planning for three weekly sessions. All the clinicians underwent training in family-focused treatment and in enhanced care during a 2-day workshop, followed with monthly supervision.

The subjects were between 12 and 18 years old and were diagnosed with bipolar I or II based on the Schedule for Affective Disorders and Schizophrenia for School-Age Children–Present and Lifetime Version. All youth had experienced manic, hypomanic, or depressive symptoms in 3 months before the study. The study concluded that participants in the family-focused treatment group showed a lower number of weeks with mania and hypomania symptoms after year 1 compared with the enhanced care group (**Fig. 2**).[10] However, family-focused treatment did not result in reduced depressive episodes.

Parent Involvement in Treatment of Disruptive Disorders

Treatment of disruptive behavior disorders, such as oppositional defiant disorder and conduct disorder, requires inclusion of support for improved parenting because the style of parenting is a risk factor for developing and maintaining these disorders. Attention-deficit/hyperactivity disorder (ADHD) is a neurodevelopmental condition that also has a behavioral component because of increased hyperactivity and impulsivity. Often negative feedback from parents and other authority figures results in progression from ADHD symptoms to more oppositional behaviors. Furlong and colleagues[25] evaluated the effectiveness of parent management training and other parenting programs in a review of RCTs of behavioral and cognitive behavioral group-based parenting programs for early onset conduct or oppositional problems in children aged 3 to 12 years. Most of the studies compared the different family intervention programs with a waiting-list group. The authors reviewed 12 studies, five from the United States (four in Seattle) and seven from Europe (three in the United Kingdom).

The number of participants per study ranged from 28 to 153; all together there were 1078 participants. Out of 1078 participants, 646 received an intervention and 432 were in the control group. Participants were predominately white with involvement of the primary caretaker alone or both parents. Average age of the parents was 33 years with 8 to 12 parents per group. A total of 68.3% of the children involved were boys.

The authors only focused on group-based parenting programs that focus on collaborative learning and practicing of parenting skills. More specifically, these skills include appropriate and constructive play, praise, rewards, and discipline. The programs

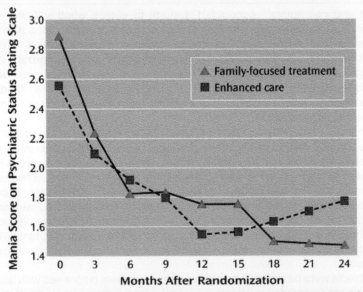

Fig. 2. Family-focused treatment versus enhanced care. (*From* Miklowitz DJ, Schneck CD, George EL, et al. Pharmacotherapy and family-focused treatment for adolescents with bipolar I and II disorders: a 2-year randomized trial. Am J Psychiatry 2014;171(6):658–67; with permission.)

reinforce the learned skills by modeling, observation, role-play, discussion, homework assignments, peer support, reframing cognitive perceptions, and addressing barriers. The frequency of these groups also ranges from 4 to 24 weekly sessions.

Nine of the 13 studies evaluated the Incredible Years BASIC Parenting Program, which consisted of videotaped vignettes of typical parent-child interactions, group discussions, role plays, and homework. Most of these programs had 9 to 16 weekly sessions that would last from 2 to 2.5 hours. Similar to these nine studies, two studies used parent management training focused on positive parenting skills. These studies evaluated programs that provided 22 to 24 weekly 2-hour sessions. For the first 10 weekly sessions, parents were taught the positive parenting skills that are encouraged further in the following five monthly sessions. One of these two programs provided additional material to manage parental stress, social support, and protective/risk factors. Similarly, the Triple P Parenting Program used the same modalities to teach positive parenting skills. However, this intervention involved four weekly 2-hour sessions with four weekly 15-minute telephone calls.

A meta-analysis was conducted of measures assessing conduct disorder, parental mental health, and parenting practices. The meta-analysis found behavioral and cognitive parent training to be effective in reducing conduct disorder behavior. The authors did not find any significant differences among the different programs evaluated. These trainings also enhanced parental mental health, thus possibly improving parent-child interactions. There is no long-term follow-up for the studies reviewed.

Multidimensional Family Therapy for Substance Abuse

MDFT was initially developed as an outpatient FBT for adolescent substance abuse.[26] It is deeply rooted in the structural family therapy model, developmental psychology, and developmental psychopathology. It is a multisystemic approach that addresses the individual characteristics of the adolescent, the parents, and the other involved family members. Additionally, it monitors and alters the interactional patterns among family members that contribute to substance abuse.[27]

Liddle[27] completed an RCT that showed the superiority of MDFT in comparison with a multifamily educational intervention (MEI) and adolescent group therapy (AGT). Participants included 13- to 18-year-old adolescents who were using illegal substances for average of 2.5 years with or without alcohol, although alcohol use was often concomitant. To confirm treatment fidelity, all three treatments were manual-guided and the sessions were videotaped. The participants were randomly assigned to one of the three treatments: MDFT, MEI, or AGT. Each arm consisted of 14 to 16 weekly sessions that occurred over 5 to 6 months. MDFT was conducted in three phases.

Similar to MDFT, MEI was also rooted in family therapy, but it integrated psychoeducational features and addressed three to four families at a time. In MEI group, didactic presentation, intrafamily or interfamily group discussion, and skill building exercises were conducted in three-part 90-minute sessions. The AGT arm had four phases that were modeled after Beck's group therapy model.[28,29] The initial phase included two family sessions to enlist family cooperation and discuss group rules. Additionally, individual meetings occurred with each adolescent to introduce the group therapy process and gather personal history. Treatment focused on skill-building by specifically focusing on drug-refusal, conflict resolution, and anger management skills. AGT concluded with generalization and maintenance of newly learned skills and relapse prevention.

The outcome of this study was measured by symptom improvement, academic performance, family competency, and increase in protective factors. These measurements were taken at the intake of the treatment, termination of the treatment, and

6- and 12-month follow-up. There was overall improvement among each treatment modality. On review of frequency of drug use, improvement in grade point average, and competency in family functioning, MDFT showed the most improvement. AGT was second best, with MEI being the last. MDFT showed rapid reductions in drug use that were maintained during the 6- and 12-month follow-ups. There was significant improvement in family functioning in the MDFT group, whereas there was no change in the AGT group and significant deterioration in MEI. The participants of the AGT group had as low frequency of drug use as those in the MDFT group after 1 year. Thus, it seems that the impact of the AGT treatment occurs over time, in comparison with the MDFT group. However, the caveat here is that there were a higher number of drop-outs in the AGT group (48%). The drop-out rate in the MDFT group was 30%, whereas it was 34% in the MEI group. This may also indicate the role a family plays in adherence to a treatment plan because the two groups with family involvement have lower drop-out rates.

Multisystemic Therapy and Functional Family Therapy for Delinquent Behavior

A meta-analysis was conducted by Baldwin and colleagues[30] to identify the best family treatment of adolescent delinquency and substance abuse. They evaluated the outcome of promising family therapy–based treatments, such as brief-strategic family therapy, functional family therapy (FFT), MDFT, and multisystemic therapy (MST), as compared with treatment as usual, alternative therapy, and control condition. Alternative treatment included group therapy, psychodynamic family therapy, individual therapy, parent groups, and family education therapy. After reviewing 24 studies, all four therapies had better outcomes than treatment as usual or alternative therapy.

MST includes elements of Minuchin's structural family therapy, Haley's strategic perspective, social learning theory, and cognitive behavioral therapy (CBT). Thus, MST hopes to address repeated patterns of interaction among family members, the behavioral impact of family hierarchy, the importance of modeling and reinforcement, and the benefit of problem-solving skills to decrease adolescent delinquency and substance abuse (discussed in more detail elsewhere in this issue).[31]

In 1995 and 2005, Borduin and colleagues[32] showed effectiveness of MST when it was applied to a sample of chronic and violent juvenile offenders. The result was that at 14-year follow-up, MST improved family relations, decreased caregiver and adolescent mental health symptoms, and decreased repetitive incarcerations by more than 50%.[33] This research was replicated to assess the effectiveness of MST with juvenile sex offenders. As expected, at 9-year follow-up, MST reduced recidivism by 83% and decreased incarcerated days by 80%.[22] In conclusion, there is sufficient evidence for MST to be an effective treatment of youth, including African-American and multiracial Hawaiian, with antisocial behavior.

FFT sees behavioral and psychiatric problems to be a result of dysfunctional family relations. Thus, FFT establishes new patterns of family interaction by integrating behavioral and cognitive strategies with direct intervention with the family.[22] In FFT, a team is composed of three to eight therapists who carry a caseload of 12 to 15 families. The treatment involves 12 sessions, which are divided in three phases over 3 to 4 months. The theme of phase 1 is engagement and motivation. The focus of phase 2 is to replace the old relational patters with more adaptive family interactions. The therapist may use other evidence-based interventions to create behavioral change. For example, CBT may be used to address the adolescent depression. Therapists may also use other problem-solving and pragmatic techniques to improve communication among family members. The goal of phase 3 is to generalize the new learned patterns and skills to the broader community.[34,35] The therapist also helps the family anticipate and plan for future barriers in sustaining positive relationships.[36]

Alexander and Parsons[23] showed the effectiveness of FFT in improving family interactions and decreasing recidivism for adolescents with status offenses. Similar to MST, the reduction in youth recidivism was significantly associated with therapist's adherence to the protocol and with increased supportive communication in families.[37] Additionally, treatment completion was associated with improvement in relationship skills among family members.[37]

Multidimensional Treatment Foster Care

Multidimensional treatment foster care (MTFC) was first developed for 12 to 17 year olds in foster care who failed intensive in-home and out-of-home services.[37] MTFC is rooted in social learning theory and natural contextual reinforcement. The promotion of prosocial behavior requires intense foster parent supervision, engagement in prosocial peer activities, removal from deviant peers, and encouragement for positive school performance. The goal is to keep this youth out of state detention centers or group care facilities.[38]

The team for MTFC is composed of a trained foster parent, a program supervisor, family therapist, individual therapist, skill trainer, and recruiter. The program supervisor is available for 24-hour crisis management. Foster parents receive 20-hour training to provide close supervision and highly structured behavior management. The caseload of the team is no more than 10 youths. Compared with MST, MDFT, and FFT, the duration of treatment usually lasts longer, on average 6 to 9 months. Family therapy, individual therapy, and skills training can continue for an additional 3 months.

The outcome of this intensive treatment was reduction in criminal charges and 60% fewer incarceration days at 1-year follow-up for chronic juvenile offenders.[39] This result was sustained at 2-year follow-up according to Eddy and coworkers.[40] The MTFC trial was further successfully generalized to adolescent female chronic offenders. The results of the study showed reduced pregnancies at 2-year follow-up.[41]

PROMISING TREATMENTS

Natural disasters, such as Hurricane Katrina, displace families from their homes and communities. While parents are trying to stabilize their lives and focus on surviving, their attention may not be on supervising their children or processing loss with their adolescents. Thus, youth in disaster-stricken areas are particularly vulnerable to mental health issues, such as PTSD. Recognizing the multifactorial postdisaster problems and the already existing evidence for MDFT, Rowe and Liddle[42] plan to generalize MDFT treatment to help adolescents with substance abuse and trauma post–Hurricane Katrina in the New Orleans region. In this RCT, they hope to compare MDFT with CBT-influenced high-quality group treatment of 13 to 17 years olds who have mild to moderate trauma symptoms and substance abuse problems.

Pineda and Dadds[43] compared a strength-based family education program called the Resourceful Adolescent Parent Program (RAP-P) with routine care (control group) when treating suicidal adolescents ages 12 to 17 years. These adolescents experienced at least one episode of suicidal behavior, which includes suicidal ideation, intent, attempt, self-injurious behavior, and parasuicidal gestures, in the previous 2 months. RAP-P is an interactive psychoeducation program for parents conducted over four 2-hour sessions. The first session identifies parental strengths and stress management strategies. The following three sessions involve education about normal adolescent development, how to promote adolescent self-esteem, how to encourage autonomy while building attachment, and managing family conflict. Of the 40 families, the families in the RAP-P group had improved family functioning and reduced adolescent suicidality after intervention and at 6-month follow-up.

Family interventions are not limited to mental health issues. There are a few non-RCT studies that evaluate family interventions to manage childhood obesity. Initially family intervention was limited to education about healthy lifestyle and exercise.[31,44,45] Epstein and colleagues[44] reviewed 10 years of data that indicate maintenance of weight can be achieved through a family-based approach. Education about parenting and parenting styles was added to a behavioral approach that showed a positive outcome over 7 years.[46,47] Kitzman-Ulrich and coworkers[48] developed a treatment model that drew from family systems theory and combined it with a behavioral approach. This treatment builds nurturance, family cohesion, and conflict resolution.[47,48] Building family competence, satisfaction, and warmth also was included. Given the positive outcome in family interventions for childhood obesity, educating the family about healthy lifestyles and improving parenting should be considered standard treatment of childhood obesity.

FURTHER RESEARCH

Although the RCTs mentioned here support using family interventions for child and adolescent mental health issues, there continues to be a need for further research. It is not yet known which treatment is best for individual families. It is also not known which treatment is indicated for varying degrees of severity of the problem. Because most psychiatric conditions have comorbidity, it would be beneficial to have data on effectiveness for comorbid conditions.

From this review, it is apparent that family interventions are effective in treating child and adolescent mental illness. However, data are needed regarding which specific interventions with the family make the difference and produce the improved outcome. Is modeling adaptive behavior sufficient to result in improved anxiety? Is psychoeducation for the family about depression the primary factor that results in improved symptomatology? The growing diversity of society requires more RCTs with a higher proportion of minority families to guide treatment of families from varying cultures. Finally, studies that examine the inclusion of the common factors listed previously in manualized treatments would further guide and refine practice.

REFERENCES

1. Sanford M, Boyle M, McCleary L, et al. A pilot study of adjunctive family psychoeducation in adolescent major depression: feasibility and treatment effect. J Am Acad Child Adolesc Psychiatry 2006;45:386–95.
2. Aman MG, McDougle CJ, Scahill L, et al. Medication and parent training in children with pervasive developmental disorders and serious behavior problems. J Am Acad Child Adolesc Psychiatry 2009;48:1143–54.
3. Handen BL, Johnson CR, Lecavalier L, et al. Use of a direct observational measure in a trial of risperidone and parent training in children and pervasive development disorders. J Dev Phys Disabil 2013;25(3):355–71.
4. Kaslow NJ, Deering CG, Racusin GR. Depressed children and their families. Clin Psychol Rev 1994;14:39–59.
5. Sheeber L, Hops H, Davis B. Family processes in adolescent depression. Clin Child Fam Psychol Rev 2001;4:19–35.
6. Diamond GS, Siqueland L. Family therapy for the treatment of depressed adolescents. Psychotherapy 1995;32:77–90.

7. Diamond GS, Reis BF, Diamond GM, et al. Attachment-based family therapy for depressed adolescents: a treatment development study. J Am Acad Child Adolesc Psychiatry 2002;41:1190–6.

8. Greenberg MT, Cicchetti D, editors. Attachment in the preschool years: theory, research, and intervention. Chicago: University of Chicago Press; 1990. p. 339–72.

9. Rudolph KD, Constance H, Burge D, et al. Toward an interpersonal life-stress model of depression: the developmental context of stress generation. Dev Psychopathol 2000;12:215–34.

10. Miklowitz DJ, Schneck CD, George EL, et al. Pharmacotherapy and family-focused treatment for adolescents with bipolar I and II disorders: a 2-year randomized trial. Am J Psychiatry 2014;171(6):658–67.

11. Diamond GS, Wintersteen MB, Brown GK, et al. Attachment-based family therapy for adolescents with suicidal ideation: a randomized controlled trial. J Am Acad Child Adolesc Psychiatry 2010;49(2):122–31.

12. Ginsburg GS, Schlossberg MC. Family-based treatment of childhood anxiety disorders. Int Rev Psychiatry 2002;14:143–54.

13. Hirshfeld DR, Biederman J, Brody L, et al. Associations between expressed emotion and child behavioral inhibition and psychopathology: a pilot study. J Am Acad Child Adolesc Psychiatry 1997;36:205–13.

14. Rapee RM. Potential role of childrearing practices in the development of anxiety and depression. Clin Psychol Rev 1997;17:47–67.

15. Kendall PC, Hudson JL, Gosch E, et al. Cognitive-behavioral therapy for anxiety disordered youth: a randomized clinical trial evaluating child and family modalities. J Consult Clin Psychol 2008;76(2):282–97.

16. Kendall PC, Hedtke KA. Coping cat workbook. 2nd edition. Ardmore (PA): Workbook; 2006.

17. Deblinger E, Heflin AH. Treating sexually abused children and their nonoffending parents: a cognitive behavioral approach. Thousand Oaks (CA): Sage Publications; 1996.

18. Cohen JA, Mannarino AP. Interventions for sexually abused children: initial treatment findings. Child Maltreat 1998;3:17–26.

19. Deblinger E, Mannarino AP, Cohen JA, et al. A follow-up study of a multisite, randomized controlled trial for children with sexual abuse-related PTSD symptoms. J Am Acad Child Adolesc Psychiatry 2006;45(12):1474–84.

20. Cohen JA, Mannarino AP. A treatment outcome study for sexually abused preschool children: initial findings. J Am Acad Child Adolesc Psychiatry 1996;35: 42–50.

21. Cohen JA, Deblinger E, Mannarino AP. Trauma-focused cognitive-behavioral therapy for sexually abused children. Psychiatr Times 2004;21(10).

22. Borduin CM, Schaeffer CM, Heiblum N. A randomized clinical trial of multi systemic therapy with juvenile sexual offenders: effects on youth social ecology and criminality activity. J Consulting Clinic Psychol 2009;77:26–37.

23. Alexander JF, Parsons BV. Short-term behavioral intervention with delinquent families: impact on family process and recidivism. J Abnormal Psychol 1973;81: 219–25.

24. Lock J, Le Grange D, Agras WS, et al. Randomized clinical trial comparing family-based treatment to adolescent focused individual therapy for adolescents with anorexia nervosa. Arch Gen Psychiatry 2010;67(10):1025–32.

25. Furlong M, McGilloway S, Bywater T, et al. Cochrane review: behavioural and cognitive-behavioural group-based parenting programmes for early-onset

conduct problems in children aged 3 to 12 years. Evid Based Child Health 2012; 2:318–692.

26. Liddle HA. Multidimensional Family Therapy Treatment (MDFT) for the Adolescent Cannabis users; Cannabis Youth Treatment (CYT) manual series. Rockville (MD): US Department of Health and Human Services; 2001. Vol. 5.

27. Liddle HA, Dakof GA, Parker K, et al. Multidimensional family therapy for adolescent drug abuse: results of a randomized clinical trial. Am J Drug Alcohol Abuse 2001;27(4):651–88.

28. Beck AP. A study of group phase development and emergent leadership. Group 1981;5(4):48–54.

29. Dugo JM, Beck AP. A therapist's guide to issues of intimacy and hostility viewed as group-level phenomena. Int J Group Psychother 1984;34:25–45.

30. Baldwin SA, Christian S, Berkeljon A, et al. The effects of family therapies for adolescent delinquency and substance abuse: a meta-analysis. J Marital Fam Ther 2012;38(1):281–304.

31. Brownell KD, Kelman JH, Stunkard AJ. Treatment of obese children with and without their mothers: changes in weight and blood pressure. Pediatrics 1983; 71:515–23.

32. Borduin CM, Mann BJ, Cone LT, et al. Multisystemic treatment of serious juvenile offenders: long term prevention of criminality and violence. J Consulting Clinic Psychol 1995;63:569–78.

33. Schaeffer CM, Borduin CM. Long-term follow up to a randomized clinical trial of multi systemic therapy with serious and violent juvenile offenders. J Consulting Clinic Psychol 2005;73:445–53.

34. Alexander JF, Parsons BV. Functional family therapy: principles and procedures. Carmel (CA): Brooks/Cole; 1982.

35. Alexander JF, Bartom C, Gordon D, et al. Blueprints for violence prevention: functional family therapy. Boulder (CO): Venture; 1998.

36. Weisz JR, Kazdin AE, editors. Evidence-based psychotherapies for children and adolescents. 2nd edition. New York: Guilford Press; 2010. p. 401–15.

37. Henggeler SW, Sheidow AJ. Empirically supported family-based treatments for conduct disorder and delinquency in adolescents. J Marital Fam Ther 2012; 38(1):30–58.

38. Alexander JF, Barton C, Schiavo RS, et al. Behavioral intervention with families of delinquents: therapist characteristics, family behavior, and outcome. J Consulting Clinic Psychol 1976;44:656–64.

39. Chamberlain P. Treating chronic juvenile offenders: advances made through the Oregon multidimensional treatment foster care model. Washington, DC: American Psychological Association; 2003.

40. Eddy JM, Whaley R, Chamberlain P. The prevention of violent behavior by chronic and serious male juvenile offenders: a 2-year follow-up of a randomized clinical trial. J Fam Psychol 2004;12:2–8.

41. Kerr DCR, Leve LD, Chamberlain P. Pregnancy rates among juvenile justice girls in two randomized controlled trials of multidimensional treatment foster care. J Consulting Clinic Psychol 2009;77:588–93.

42. Rowe CL, Liddle HA. When the levee breaks: treating adolescents and families in the aftermath of Hurricane Katrina. J Marital Fam Ther 2008;34(2):132–48.

43. Pineda J, Dadds MR. Family intervention for adolescents with suicidal behavior: a randomized controlled trial and mediation analysis. J Am Acad Child Psychiatry 2013;52(8):851–62.

44. Epstein LH, Valoski A, Wing RR, et al. Ten-year outcomes of behavioral family-based treatment for childhood obesity. Health Psychol 1994;13:373–83.
45. Israel AC, Stolmaker L, Andrian CA. The effects of training parents in general child management skills on a behavioral weight loss program for children. Behav Ther 1985;16:169–80.
46. Golan M, Weizman A, Apter A, et al. Parents as the exclusive agents of change in the treatment of childhood obesity. Am J Clin Nutr 1998;67:1130–5.
47. Golan M. Parents as agents of change in childhood obesity: from research to practice. Int J Pediatr Obes 2006;1:66–76.
48. Kitzman-Ulrich H, Hampson R, Wilson DK, et al. An adolescent weight-loss program integrating family variables reduces energy intake. J Am Diet Assoc 2009; 109:491–6.

The Family Couch
Considerations for Infant/Early Childhood Mental Health

Susan Dickstein, PhD

KEYWORDS

- Infant/early childhood • Mental health • Family • Stress

KEY POINTS

- Infant/early childhood mental health is defined as "the young child's capacity to experience, regulate and express emotions; form close and secure interpersonal relationships; explore and act on the environment and learn…(that is) best accomplished within the context of the caregiving environment that includes family, community and cultural expectations."
- Infant and early childhood mental health principles and practices are inherently systems based and multigenerational, which emphasize working with and through family relationships to optimize early mental health outcomes.
- Strategies to promote infant/early childhood mental health involve simultaneous attention to characteristics of the infant or toddler, the parent, and the developing attachment relationship, all within the family, community, and cultural systems within which the young child and parents reside.

She is as in a field a silken tent
At midday when a sunny summer breeze
Has dried the dew and all its ropes relent,
So that in guys it gently sways at ease,
And its supporting central cedar pole,
That is its pinnacle to heavenward
And signifies the sureness of the soul,
Seems to owe naught to any single cord,
But strictly held by none, is loosely bound
By countless silken ties of love and thought
To everything on earth the compass round…

—Robert Frost

The author has nothing to disclose.
Bradley Hospital/Warren Alpert Medical School of Brown University, Box G-A1, Providence, RI 02912, USA
E-mail address: Susan_Dickstein@Brown.edu

Child Adolesc Psychiatric Clin N Am 24 (2015) 487–500
http://dx.doi.org/10.1016/j.chc.2015.02.004
1056-4993/15/$ – see front matter © 2015 Elsevier Inc. All rights reserved.

childpsych.theclinics.com

Abbreviations	
ABC	Attachment and Biobehavioral Catch-Up
COS	Circle of Security
CPP	Child-Parent Psychotherapy
VIPP	Video Feedback to Promote Positive Parenting

WHAT IS INFANT/EARLY CHILDHOOD MENTAL HEALTH?

The birth of the infant-family field is generally credited to Selma Fraiberg, whose pioneering work focused on promoting infant/early childhood mental health by understanding and working through the relationships that were most salient for infants and young children.[1,2] An accepted definition of infant/early childhood mental health is "the young child's capacity to experience, regulate and express emotions; form close and secure interpersonal relationships; explore and act on the environment and learn...(that is) best accomplished within the context of the caregiving environment that includes family, community and cultural expectations..."[3] Family relationships are at the core, reflecting Winnicott's[4] assertion that "there is no such thing as a child" separate from the multigenerational family experiences within which the child is raised. In this article, the power of family relationships is described as central to the continuum of infant/early childhood mental health practices, including promoting early social-emotional well-being and development, preventing adverse outcomes in the context of risk, and intervening to treat symptoms associated with mental health disorders.

Infant/Early Childhood Mental Health Challenges

Infants and very young children can evidence mental health symptoms and disorders.[5–7] Infants and young children are good at showing us when they are experiencing mental "health"—they are curious, enchanting, persistent, and confident. When they are experiencing mental health challenges, they can be listless, distracted, aggressive, or insecure. Infants and toddlers can experience grief, sadness, anger, and hopelessness, which in their extreme forms may manifest as mood and anxiety disorders, disorders of regulation (feeding, sleep, sensory, behavior), and posttraumatic stress disorder (eg, Ref.[8]). The associated social-emotional and behavior challenges affect all domains of early development, as well as the physical health, mental health, and development of the child for a lifetime (eg, Ref.[9]). Therefore, it is imperative that challenges are addressed as early as possible. But how can this be done when the child cannot independently seek out treatment and may not be able to verbally describe the pain or distress he or she might be suffering?

This dilemma calls to mind an image of an infant in diapers lying on a tiny couch with a clinician sitting nearby attempting to discover the nature of her symptoms. This article does not suggest that the image of a couch is of no use (and, in fact, it links us to the field's psychodynamic roots) but rather that the couch would need to be of the largest size possible to include everyone connected to her. That is, infant/early childhood mental health symptoms and disorders can only be understood, and addressed, in the context of current and historical family experiences into which the infant has been born and is developing. These close relationships with parents and other significant caregivers are embedded within unique interpretive frameworks (eg, cultural, historical, family values, and parenting beliefs) that serve to organize parent-infant interaction experiences.[10] In addition, because all early social-emotional development occurs in the context of relationships, the emotional well-being of the infant/young child depends on the emotional health of the child's parents and other significant care providers.[11] Thus, in addition to the characteristics and vulnerabilities of the infant, one needs to make room on the couch to consider the influence of parental characteristics (eg, depression, history of unresolved loss, or trauma), interparental and co-parenting issues, contextual factors (eg, trauma, social isolation, or poverty), and other sources of significant support or disruption as they influence the meaning parents give to the child's symptoms, as well as their capacity to be available to the young child as a committed and protective relationship partner. One also needs to make room on the couch for the parallel process that requires the therapist to be present with and for the parent to make use of the therapeutic relationship that may guide the parent to repair and strengthen his or her relationship with the young child. A very large couch indeed.

Theoretic Underpinnings

The infant-family field is rooted in core principles and practices that place the parent-child attachment relationship as central.[9,12,13] In recent years, acceptance of these foundations have been strengthened by emerging research from neuroscience on environmental and social influences on early brain development that support the critical nature of relationships and early experiences for lifelong physical and mental health.[14–17] In many ways, family systems theory and related family intervention strategies extend these roots. In particular, 2 related tenets of family systems theory are relevant.[18] First, families are composed of subsystems (smaller relationship units with different levels of organization), each with its own unique properties, interaction rules, and boundary distinctions. Second, the whole (family) is greater than the sum of its parts. As applied to infant/early childhood mental health, it is considered that (1) child development occurs in the context of multiple levels of relational systems (eg, parent-child, parent-parent, family unit) that impinge on each other; (2) not only do children change, grow, and develop over time but also family systems themselves experience transitions in structure, resources, and routines; and (3) when stressed, the complex accumulation of risk factors affects early development as well as (and perhaps through) family functioning.

Research suggests that the unique yet interlocking systems within the family are differentially related to infant developmental outcomes.[19] For example, with respect to the risk to early development posed by maternal depression, Dickstein and colleagues[20] found significant associations between (1) maternal depression and marital functioning as well as (2) maternal depression and quality of parent-child interaction. These links became less clear when the overall quality of family unit functioning was considered. That is, the nature of family (unit) functioning mediated the direct associations between the smaller subsystems.

This perspective helps to highlight the complexity of the work that individual characteristics of children, parents, and families develop over time and are changed by the series of multidirectional interactions that happen among children, parents, and the family environment. To support infant/early childhood mental health, one embraces this complexity and focuses on the regulatory mechanisms that are thought to promote change.[21,22] As Sameroff[23] states, "…several things are clear. Children affect their environments and environments affect children. Moreover, environmental settings affect and are affected by each other. These effects change over time in response to normative and non-normative events. Children are neither doomed nor protected by their own characteristics or the characteristics of the caregiver alone. The complexity…opens up the possibility for many avenues of intervention to facilitate the healthy development of infants and families."

CORE CONCEPTS IN THE INFANT-FAMILY FIELD

The goal of the infant-family field is to promote infant/early childhood mental health, prevent poor outcomes in the context of risk, and relieve psychological suffering by screening for, diagnosing (as relevant), and treating mental health disorders early in infancy and early childhood before other areas of development are affected. Social and emotional development is considered to be the cornerstone of healthy development; it provides a foundation on which all subsequent development rests, including cognitive competencies and later school success.[11,24] Because parenting confidence and competence develop in the context of the family, one focuses on the capacity of the family system to support the emotional health of all its members, as well as to provide basic resources necessary for healthy growth and development; this includes focus on the emotional health of the parent and the nature of parent-child relationships. Taken together, the family is a powerful system that has the capacity to support, nurture, and protect (or not) each parent's own mental health as the parent manages the transitions and relationship demands that come with the addition of a new baby to the family.[11]

Core Concept 1: Optimal Development Depends on Relationship Security—The Central Role of Attachment Within the Family System

Attachment is at the core of the relational framework of the infant-family field.[25,26] The way that early development unfolds is shaped both by the child's innate characteristics and traits (eg, physiologic sensitivity to stress) and the experiences the child has with relationship partners from the beginning of life. Infants and young children are biologically wired to seek out and thrive on experiences with parents and primary caregivers and depend on nurturing and secure relationships to help them develop optimally across all domains of development. That is, the attachment system is coordinated with the exploratory system. When infants and young children are engaged in exploring the world of toys, objects, or people, the attachment system is quiet (the child is not in active need of a parent's reassurance or protection). When the infant becomes stressed or distressed (hungry/fatigued, an unfamiliar adult approaches, an older sibling pulls the baby's hair, a trusted caregiver leaves the play area to check on a peer), exploration decreases as the attachment system is activated; the infant might signal that he or she is stressed by crying or reaching toward the attachment figure, and the infant might seek proximity to the parent and maintain contact until emotional equilibrium is regained. The child's temperament, in part, guides the intensity and emotionality of the stress reaction, with each child displaying a unique repertoire of stress and signaling behaviors.[27]

The parent facilitates the emotion regulation process by responding sensitively and contingently to the infant's cues and being a consistent and committed partner. As Shonkoff describes, the end result of this serve and return process is an infant who has regained emotional control and smoothly returns to the work of exploration.[28] As such, a securely attached infant not only gains experience with the power of expressing and regulating emotions but also learns to trust what he or she feels because someone is regularly there to meet the infant's needs; experiences the environment as predictable and safe; and comes to expect success in social interactions with others, a lesson that shapes the infant's approach to relationships with peers and later with adult romantic partners.

The infant is not the only one to benefit from secure serve and return interactions with parents. Secure relationships are powerful for parents as well. The parent of a securely attached infant has numerous opportunities to experience delight with the infant and confidence in parenting capacity as he or she effectively reads and responds to the child's cues and needs for nurturance and protection. When it works well, it is a system in balance.

What happens when the system is out of balance? Infants who have had repeated early parenting experiences that involve rejection of their needs or lack of contingent responsiveness are likely to develop insecure attachments with the caregiver. Infants with insecure attachments tend to have trouble regulating affect especially during stressful situations and may exhibit poor self-control or excessive anxiety. They may have trouble relying on others for comfort because their experiences have not supported that others are trustworthy stewards of their affective distress. Similarly, parents of infants with insecure attachments may feel like ineffective relationship partners, may describe their babies as difficult, and may have trouble with trust and security in adult intimate relationships themselves.

Decades of research on attachment illuminate mechanisms by which parental perceptions and expectations of relationship security influence the quality of relationships parents develop with their infants in their current family contexts.[26] Because attachment relationships influence the developing sense of self as well as the developing expectations of the extent to which others can be relied on as emotional and social supports, they have meaning across generations. That is, the parent's historical (and current adult) relationship experiences become integrated into a representational relationship framework that is transmitted within the current parent-child relationship. For example, it is known that mothers' representations of their early experiences with their own parents influence interaction patterns they develop with their children.[29-31] These internal representations have been related to capacity for affective attunement with their infants[32-34] and security of attachment.[35] Furthermore, research on relationship experiences between adult partners has been found to predict security within that relationship (eg, Refs.[36-38]). Higher-quality marital and/or co-parenting relationships are associated with more positive parenting behavior as well as more positive parent-child relationships.[39]

Although patterns of attachment can be carried forward into the next generation, "history is not destiny."[2] When a new baby joins the family, the family system adjusts by coordinating multiple roles, tasks, and transactions across all the individuals and alliances within the family. The family system adjusts as it enters a new family developmental stage and as it interfaces with community supports that might be available and necessary. In the face of challenges, the potential for change exists by exploring how patterns might reflect a reawakening from the past that can now be considered with a fresh perspective.

Concept 2: Optimal Development Depends on Relationship Safety to Mediate Stress

Brain science has made strides that directly inform the principles and practices of the infant/family field. There is now solid evidence from the field of neuroscience that early brain development is influenced by experiences the young child has. In particular, the repeated and reciprocal back and forth exchanges within a primary relationship context (ie, serve and return mechanism described earlier) is responsible for foundational neural wiring and shaping the architecture of the young brain.[16,40,41]

Early stress experiences and attachment

One of the main functions of the attachment system is to support the infant's emerging capacity for emotion regulation, initially controlled by the parent and over time more self-controlled by the baby. This system is activated in the presence of stress. Normative levels of stress are expected and facilitate social-emotional learning (eg, when a parent separates from the child for a short time; when a child feels hungry or uncomfortable). At these times, when the child becomes stressed or distressed, the caregiver responds sensitively and contingently to the child's cues and comforts the child in a manner that relieves the stress. These repeated serve and return experiences promote the child's emerging capacity for self-regulation of arousal and emotion, a foundation for social-emotional health.[14,42]

On the other hand, toxic (or traumatic) stress that chronically occurs within the context of the child's care-giving system (such as abuse, neglect, or interparent domestic violence) or occurs outside the relationship but without the protective benefits of the primary relationship can involve prolonged activation of the stress response system that overwhelms the infant or young child. In the absence of a secure parenting relationship, the child's capacity to regulate emotional states breaks down,[43] and the serve and return functions of the primary caregiving relationship are disrupted. The developing brain reacts to physiologic and environmental threats and is changed by them (eg, Ref.[44]). For example, the experience of maltreatment during infancy and early childhood can severely compromise the baby's emerging capacities to regulate emotions and alter developmental trajectories toward poor outcomes. Infants who experience maltreatment are more likely to have core deficits in forming and engaging in secure interpersonal relationships, regulating affect, and developing positive sense of self, the very deficits that set the stage for later school failure and juvenile delinquency.[12]

The brain is wired such that early learning is the foundation for later learning. For example, early traumatic experiences are associated with serious physical and mental health problems throughout the life span, and early traumatic experiences change brain architecture associated with emerging social-emotional competence, a foundation for school success. As Shonkoff and colleagues[45] at the Center on the Developing Child at Harvard indicate, "the brain's capacity for change decreases with age...It is easier and more effective to influence a baby's developing brain architecture than to rewire parts of its circuitry...(later on)." So, although a baby does not have the memory and language capacity to describe his or her experience, it gets wired into his or her physiology and brain architecture.

Behavioral epigenetics research has become influential in the development of new conceptual models that have implications for intervention in the area of infant/early childhood mental health[15]; further discussion on behavioral epigenetics is beyond the scope of this article. General aspects of stress and relational functioning are discussed as relevant for family work with infants/young children and their families. For example, Lillis and Turnbull[46,47] developed the Neurorelational Framework that considers the infant and young child and parent's individual neurodevelopmental differences with respect to 4 brain system capacities (regulation, sensory, relevance, and executive) that mirror the complexity of the family's presenting challenges and quality of parent-child engagement. Stress experiences and stress recovery patterns are also considered (including overreactivity, repeated reactivity, prolonged reactivity, and chronic reactivity), and derived patterns are beginning to be used to support parent-infant relational functioning.

Core Concept 3: Working Through Relationships to Promote Infant/Early Childhood Mental Health

A unique aspect of the infant-family field is the intentional work within the parent-child relationship. Promoting well-being, preventing poor outcomes in the context of risk, and treating early childhood mental health challenges are conducted through the lens of the rich attachment relationship patterns within the child's family.[10] Further, research suggests that, to optimize early outcomes, families need to be supported before problems arise or before challenges more broadly disrupt developmental and relational functioning.

To this end, Bakermans-Kranenburg and colleagues[48] conducted a meta-analysis of 70 studies describing 88 interventions designed to enhance parenting sensitivity or security of infant attachment. The researchers concluded that highly focused programs that specifically target parenting sensitivity were effective in improving insensitive maternal behavior as well as improving rates of insecure parent-infant attachment. The following are the findings.

First, better outcomes with respect to parenting sensitivity and security of attachment were achieved for interventions that involved fewer contacts (less than 16 sessions), that started at 6 months after birth or later, and that involved the use of video feedback techniques. It is possible that shorter-term interventions were more precisely defined to target the outcomes of interest that (from a research perspective) may be more amenable to examination after the second half of the first year of the child's life. Moreover, it is possible that with fewer sessions, it is easier (for both the family and the practitioner) to sustain regular and consistent participation. Further, use of video feedback techniques (review of videotaped interactions of the actual parent-child dyad) may enhance personalization by providing opportunity for the parent to reflect on what is seen in the video as well as what might be represented, both of which (when sensitively handled) serve as a basis for trust between the parent and practitioner.

Second, risk characteristics of the sample did not tend to be associated with effectiveness of the intervention. That is, even parents who experienced more contextual burdens showed improvement in parenting sensitivity. Clinical samples (ie, those identified with diagnosed challenges such as maternal depression) did better than their nonclinical counterparts.

Finally, the research suggested that interventions that included fathers (in addition to mothers) were more effective than those that focused only on mothers; this speaks to the powerful influence of family systems mechanisms for improving parent-child relationship quality. Infants and young children's mental health depends not only on a secure relationship with the mother but also on supportive relationships that exist between the important adults who care for and are committed to the infant's well-being.[49]

RELATIONSHIP-BASED STRATEGIES TO PROMOTE INFANT/EARLY CHILDHOOD MENTAL HEALTH

Creating the right conditions for infant/early childhood mental health is a critical path to prevent the need to address child problems later on. One of the most important mediators for infant/early childhood mental health outcomes in the context of developmental risk is the quality of the parent-child attachment relationship in all its contextual complexity.[50] Thus, practitioners in the infant-family field work to prevent early mental health challenges by actively enhancing early parent-child relationships that develop in the context of stress.[28] Strategies to promote infant/early childhood mental health involve simultaneous attention to characteristics of the infant or toddler, the parent, and the developing attachment relationship[11]; this is understood only within the family, community, and cultural systems within which the young child and parents reside. When social, emotional, sensory, or regulatory challenges (or disorders) are identified early on, assessment and treatment ports of entry are considered at all levels of the family system, including (but not necessarily limited to) provision of emotional support to parents, concrete resource assistance, developmental guidance, and psychotherapeutic intervention that addresses the needs of relationships vis-à-vis infant/early childhood mental health challenges. **Table 1** describes essential

Table 1
Levels of family functioning related to promotion of infant/early childhood mental health

Level of Family	Factors to Consider to Promote Infant/Early Childhood Mental Health
Who is this infant/young child?	What are unique characteristics of this child considered to be developmental strengths and vulnerabilities? In what ways does the infant/young child express, experience, and regulate emotions to signal his or her needs? What kind of care does this particular child require? In what ways does this child seek out and accept comfort from a parent when upset?
Who is this parent in relation to this child?	What developmental strengths and vulnerabilities are unique characteristics of this parent? Is the parent's physical and mental health a source of support or stress for the infant/young child? How confident does the parent feel about his or her capacity to care for this particular child at this time? How does the parent understand his or her own past experiences? In what ways do the parent's important adult relationships affect his or her capacity to parent this child?
Who is this parent-child dyad?	What unique strengths and vulnerabilities are characteristics of this dyad? What is the nature of the parent-child relationship? Are expectations that each has of the other generally met? Does the dyad seem to fit well together with respect to intensity, consistency, or nature of regulatory patterns?
Who is this family?	What unique strengths and vulnerabilities are characteristics of this family as a unit? Who is in the family (and who is out)? What co-parenting alliances exist to support infant/early childhood mental health? What gets in the way of supportive co-parenting? Does the family structure support safety and security within the parent-child relationship? What family routines, values, and cultural beliefs and practices guide parenting this child?
Who is beyond the family?	What are the unique characteristics of this community considered to be resources or sources of vulnerability for the family? How do extended family, community, and cultural factors affect the family's capacity to support the healthy development of the child? How are other natural (and professional) supports accessed by the family to facilitate promotion of healthy family relationships?

Data from Refs.[51–53]

targets at various levels of the family system that must be considered to effectively assess and address infant/early childhood mental health challenges.[51–53]

Attachment-Specific Interventions

Practitioners who provide clinical supports to treat infant/early childhood mental health challenges are required to attend to multiple levels of the family system to support the safety and security of the parent-child relationship. In general, work is done with parents who are encouraged:

1. To recognize and embrace the critical importance of their role in the return side of the serve and return process, that is, to support the parent to comfort the young child when the child is stressed or distressed and to facilitate the young child's active exploration of the world by creating a safe environment free from physical and emotional toxins
2. To understand early social-emotional development from the perspective of their infant/young child and to interpret the young child's behaviors and emotions within an appropriate developmental context
3. To express and reflect on their own strengths and limitations that they bring to the relationship with the child, as well as their own histories, experiences, and expectations that have shaped them as parents
4. To discover (or rediscover) feelings of delight in their child by gaining confidence to observe, understand, and protect this child, even in the face of challenges
5. To identify and collaborate with community resources that might be required to support healthy family functioning, such as provision of basic security needs (eg, food, stable housing, safe family and community circumstances), treatment of adult mental health challenges that affect parenting (such as depression and substance use), and ongoing assessment of infant disorders and disabilities, as necessary

Several intervention strategies to promote infant/early childhood mental health have emerged from attachment theoretic origins. Although they differ in the specific elements emphasized as part of the intervention protocol and methods used, they all work toward enhancing the characteristics described earlier. Four of these strategies are briefly described later, including Video Feedback Intervention to Promote Positive Parenting (VIPP), Circle of Security (COS), Attachment and Biobehavioral Catch-Up (ABC), and Child-Parent Psychotherapy (CPP).

VIPP is a home-based parent-child attachment-focused intervention. Developed by Van Ijzendoorn and colleagues,[54] it is based on their work conducted with high-risk families with children as young as 4 months of age. This strategy is based on interaction guidance techniques that have been proved effective for engaging with high-risk and overburdened families.[55] VIPP specifically promotes positive parenting by enhancing parental sensitivity and responsiveness to children's cues, increasing parental empathy, and improving the quality of parent-child interactions.[48]

ABC[56,57] is a 10-session home-based intervention designed to treat children in foster care settings whose circumstances involve significant relationship disruption including separations from primary attachment figures with concomitant issues related to eliciting and accepting (or not) care and nurturance from a new caregiver. Intervention components include the use of a trained coach to (1) help the foster parent understand the child's need and unique signals for nurturance, (2) support the foster parent to respond in a sensitive manner especially to the child's signals of distress, and (3) target behavioral, emotional, and neuroendocrine dysregulation in the child by supporting the foster parent to allow the child to both express and gain mastery over strong (and often overwhelming) emotions. Results suggest that young children whose foster parents participated with them in the ABC intervention showed less avoidance of nurturing care and more typical daily patterns of cortisol production than foster children who did not receive this treatment.

COS[58,59] is a 20-week group-based parent early education and clinical treatment model that is designed to help parents specifically provide 2 components of a secure attachment relationship, that is, a secure base and a safe haven for their children.

Results have shown that parents demonstrate enhanced relationship capacity to provide nurturance and support to their children.

CPP[60–63] is an empirically supported, relationship-based treatment of children birth to 5 years of age and their primary parenting figures, conducted in a clinical treatment setting. CPP is a dyadic and relationship-based treatment model that uses the attachment relationship as the vehicle to address early mental health challenges related to stress, trauma, and the parenting problems associated with these issues. CPP is multitheoretical in its approach, using attachment, psychoanalytic, development, and trauma theory through a cultural lens to understand and treat the family. Research has shown that CPP helps to reduce child and maternal mental health symptoms, enhance parent-child relationships and attachment security, and improve child cognitive functioning.

SUMMARY

Family systems work extends the influence of parent-child attachment beyond the emphasis on continuity and stability of working models, across time and across generations, to develop interventions used in real-world settings. It fosters consideration of the developmental life of the family per se, including important family stages and transitions, unique family membership at different points in time, and particular circumstances that influence the family at various times. Family systems work provides mechanisms for stimulating change in relationship dynamics to improve individual, subsystem, and family unit functioning. Advancements in infant-family mental health, including important contribution from neuroscience, have set the stage for the understanding that to best promote early development, assessment protocols must examine relationship complexity in the family. One should understand the nature of individual child and parent characteristics and neurodevelopmental capacities, parent-child relationships, adult-adult relationship (eg, marital, co-parenting, and parent-grandparent), and family-unit capacities for supporting the emerging social and emotional health of infants, young children, and their important caregivers. This important foundation sets the stage for lifelong mental health and well-being.

REFERENCES

1. Fraiberg S, Adelson E, Shapiro V. Ghosts in the nursery: a psychoanalytic approach to the problems of impaired infant-parent relationships. J Am Acad Child Adolesc Psychiatry 1975;14:387–421.
2. Fraiberg S. Every child's birthright: in defense of mothering. New York: Basic Books; 1977.
3. Zeanah CH, Zeanah PD. Toward a definition of infant mental health. Zero to Three 2001;22:13–20.
4. Winnicott D. The Child, the Family, and the Outside World. Harmondsworth, UK: Penguin Books; 1964.
5. Egger HL, Angold A. Common emotional and behavioral disorders in preschool children: presentation, nosology, and epidemiology. J Child Psychol Psychiatry 2006;47(3–4):313–37.
6. Gleason MM, Zeanah CH, Dickstein S. Recognizing young children in need of mental health assessment: development and preliminary validity of the early childhood screening assessment. Infant Ment Health J 2010;31(3):1–22.
7. Papousek M, Schieche M, Wurmser H. Disorders of behavioral and emotional regulation in the first years of life: early risks and intervention in the developing parent-infant relationship. Washington, DC: Zero to Three Press; 2007.

8. Northcutt C, McCarroll B. DC:0-3: a diagnostic schema for infants and young children and their families. In: Brandt K, Perry BD, Seligman S, et al, editors. Infant and early childhood mental health: core concepts and clinical practice. Washington, DC: American Psychiatric Publishing; 2014. p. 175–93 Chapter 11.

9. Hinshaw SP, Joubert CL. Developmental psychopathology: core principles and implications for child mental health. In: Brandt K, Perry BD, Seligman S, et al, editors. Infant and early childhood mental health: core concepts and clinical practice. Washington, DC: American Psychiatric Publishing; 2014. p. 249–60 Chapter 16.

10. Sameroff AJ, Fiese BH. Transactional regulation and early intervention. In: Meisels SJ, Shonkoff JP, editors. Handbook of early childhood intervention. 2nd edition. New York: Cambridge University Press; 2000. p. 119–49.

11. Weatherston DJ. The gift of love: a birthright. ChildLinks (Newsletter of Michigan Association for Infant Mental Health) 2013;1–7.

12. Cicchetti D, Toth SL. The past achievements and future promises of developmental psychopathology: the coming of age of a discipline. J Child Psychol Psychiatry 2009;50:16–25.

13. Sameroff AJ. Models of development and developmental risk. In: Zeanah CH, editor. Handbook of infant mental health. New York: Guilford Press; 1993. p. 3–13.

14. Fox SE, Levitt P, Nelson CA 3rd. How the timing and quality of early experiences influence the development of brain architecture. Child Dev 2010;81:28–40.

15. Lester BM, Marsit CJ, Bromer BS. Behavioral epigenetics and the developmental origins of child mental health disorders. In: Brandt K, Perry BD, Seligman S, et al, editors. Infant and early childhood mental health: core concepts and clinical practice. Washington, DC: American Psychiatric Publishing; 2014. p. 161–73 Chapter 10.

16. Patterson JE, Vakili S. Relationships, environment, and the brain: how emerging research is changing what we know about the impact of families on human development. Fam Process 2014;53(1):22–32.

17. Shonkoff JP. Building a new biodevelopmental framework to guide the future of early childhood policy. Child Dev 2010;81:357–67.

18. Minuchin P. Families and individual development: provocations from the field of family therapy. Child Dev 1985;56:289–302.

19. Hayden L, Schiller M, Dickstein S, et al. Levels of family assessment I: family, marital, and parent-child interaction. J Fam Psychol 1998;12:7–22.

20. Dickstein S, Hayden LC, Schiller M, et al. Levels of family assessment II: family functioning and parental psychopathology. J Fam Psychol 1998;12:23–40.

21. Bronfenbrenner U. Toward an experimental ecology of human development. Am Psychol 1977;32:513–31.

22. National Research Council, Institute of Medicine. From neurons to neighborhoods: the science of early childhood development In: Shonkoff JP, Phillips DA, editors. Washington, DC: National Academy Press; 2000.

23. Sameroff AJ. The transactional model. In: Sameroff AJ, editor. The transactional model of development: how children and contexts shape each other. Washington, DC: American Psychological Association; 2009. p. 3–21.

24. Zeanah CH, Zeanah PD. The scope of infant mental health. In: Zeanah CH, editor. Handbook of infant mental health. 3rd edition. New York: Guilford Press; 2009. p. 5–22 Chapter 1.

25. Bowlby J. Attachment and loss, volume. I: attachment. New York: Basic Books; 1982.

26. Cassidy J, Shaver PR. Handbook of attachment: theory, research and clinical applications. New York: Guilford Press; 2008.
27. Vaughn BE, Bost KK, van IJZendoorn MH. Attachment and temperament: additive and interactive influences on behavior, affect, and cognition during infancy and childhood. In: Cassidy J, Shaver PR, editors. Handbook of attachment: theory, research and clinical applications. New York: Guilford Press; 2008. p. 192–216 Chapter 9.
28. The Science of Early Childhood Development. National Scientific Council on the Developing Child. 2007. Available at: http://developingchild.net. Accessed February 18, 2015.
29. Dickstein S, Seifer R, Albus KE. Maternal adult attachment representations across relationship domains and infant outcomes: the importance of family and couple functioning. Attachment & Human Development 2009;11(1):5–27.
30. George C, Kaplan N, Main M. Adult attachment interview. Berkeley (CA): University of California at Berkeley; 1985.
31. George C, Kaplan N, Main M. Adult attachment interview. Berkeley (CA): University of California at Berkeley; 1996.
32. Benoit D, Zeanah CH, Barton ML. Maternal attachment disturbances in failure to thrive. Infant Ment Health J 1989;3:185–202.
33. Benoit D, Zeanah CH, Boucher C, et al. Sleep disorders in early childhood: association with insecure maternal attachment. J Am Acad Child Adolesc Psychiatry 1989;31(1):86–93.
34. Crowell JA, Feldman SS. Mothers' working models of attachment relationships and mother and child behavior during separation and reunion. Dev Psychol 1991;27:597–605.
35. Seifer R, Sameroff AJ, Dickstein S, et al. Parental psychopathology, multiple contextual risks, and one-year outcomes in children. J Clin Child Psychol 1996; 25:423–35.
36. Dickstein S, Seifer R, St. Andre M, et al. Marital attachment interview: adult attachment assessment of marriage. J Soc Pers Relat 2001;18(5):651–72.
37. Dickstein S. Marital attachment narratives and family functioning. In: Fiese BF, Pratt M, editors. Family stories and life course: across time and generations. NJ: Lawrence Erlbaum Assoc., Inc; 2004. p. 213–32.
38. Veroff J, Sutherland L, Chadiha LA, et al. Predicting marital quality with narrative assessments of marital experience. J Marriage Fam 1993;55:326–37.
39. McHale J, Fivaz-Depeursinge E, Dickstein S, et al. New evidence for the social embeddedness of infants early triangular capacities. Fam Process 2008;47:445–63.
40. Brandt K. Core concepts in infant-family and early childhood mental health. In: Brandt K, Perry BD, Seligman S, et al, editors. Infant and early childhood mental health: core concepts and clinical practice. Washington, DC: American Psychiatric Publishing; 2014. p. 1–20 Chapter 1.
41. Center on the Developing Child, Harvard University. Available at: www.developingchild.harvard.edu. Accessed February 18, 2015.
42. Salisbury AL, High P, Chapman H, et al. A randomized control trial of integrated care for families managing infant colic. Infant Ment Health J 2012;33:110–22.
43. van der Kolk B. Developmental trauma disorder: towards a rational diagnosis for children with complex trauma histories. Psychiatr Ann 2005;35:401–8.
44. Perry BD. The neurosequential model of therapeutics. In: Brandt K, Perry BD, Seligman S, et al, editors. Infant and early childhood mental health: core concepts and clinical practice. Washington, DC: American Psychiatric Publishing; 2014. p. 21–53 Chapter 2.

45. Shonkoff, J, Center on the Developing Child at Harvard University. A Science-Based Framework for Early Childhood Policy: Using Evidence to Improve Outcomes in Learning, Behavior, and Health for Vulnerable Children; 2007. Available at: http://www.developingchild.harvard.edu. Accessed February 18, 2015.
46. Lillas C. The neurorelational framework in infant and early childhood mental health. In: Brandt K, Perry BD, Seligman S, et al, editors. Infant and early childhood mental health: core concepts and clinical practice. Washington, DC: American Psychiatric Publishing; 2014. p. 85–95 Chapter 5.
47. Lillas C, Turnbull J. Infant/Child mental health, early intervention, and relationship-based therapies: a neurorelational framework for interdisciplinary practice. New York: WW Norton; 2009.
48. Bakermans-Kranenburg MJ, Van IJzendoorn MH, Juffer F. Less is more. Psychol Bull 2003;129(2):195–215.
49. McHale JP. Charting the bumpy road of co-parenthood: understanding the challenges of family life. Washington, DC: Zero to Three Press; 2007.
50. Zeanah CH, Bailey LO, Berry S. Infant mental health and the "real world" – opportunities for interface and impact. Child Adolesc Psychiatr Clin N Am 2009;18: 773–87.
51. Appleyard K, Berlin LJ. Supporting healthy relationships between young children and their parents: lessons from attachment theory and research. Durham, NC: Center for Child and Family Policy - Duke University; 2007.
52. Sameroff AJ, McDonough SC, Rosenblum KL. Treating parent-infant relationship problems: strategies for intervention. New York: Guilford Press; 2004.
53. Weatherston DJ. The infant mental health specialist. Washington, DC: Zero to Three Press; 2000. p. 3–10.
54. Juffer F, Bakerman-Krakenburg MJ, Van Ijzendoorn MH. Promoting positive parenting: an attachment-based intervention. Mahway (NJ): Lawrence Erlbaum Assoc., Inc; 2007.
55. McDonough S. Interaction guidance: promoting and nurturing the caregiving relationship. In: Sameroff AJ, MDonough S, Rosenblum K, editors. Treating parent-infant relationship problems: strategies for intervention. New York: Guilford Press; 2004. p. 79–95.
56. Dozier M, Lindheim O, Ackerman JP. Attachment and biobehavioral catch-up: an intervention targeting empirically identified needs of foster infants. In: Berlin LJ, Ziv Y, Amaya-Jackson L, et al, editors. Enhancing early attachments: theory, research, intervention, and policy. New York: Guilford Press; 2005. p. 178–94.
57. Dozier M, Rutter M. Challenges to the development of attachment relationships faced by young children in foster and adoptive care. In: Cassidy J, Shaver PR, editors. Handbook of attachment: theory, research and clinical implications. New York: Guilford Press; 2008. p. 698–717 Chapter 29.
58. Cooper G, Hoffman K, Powell B, et al. The circle of security intervention: differential diagnosis and differential treatment. In: Berlin LJ, Ziv Y, Amaya-Jackson L, et al, editors. Enhancing early attachments: theory, research, intervention, and policy. New York: Guilford Press; 2005. p. 127–51.
59. Powell B, Cooper G, Hoffman K, et al. The circle of security. In: Zeanah C, editor. Handbook of infant mental health. 3rd edition. New York: Guilford Press; 2009. p. 450–67 Chapter 28.
60. Lieberman AF. Child-parent psychotherapy: a relationship-based approach to the treatment of mental health disorders in infancy and early childhood. In: Sameroff AJ, McDonough SC, & KL Rosenblum, editors. Treating parent-infant

relationship problems: strategies for intervention. New York: Guilford Press; 2004. p. 97–122.

61. Lieberman AF, van Horn P. Don't hit my mommy: a manual for child-parent psychotherapy with young witnesses of family violence. Washington, DC: Zero to Three Press; 2005.

62. Lieberman AF, van Horn P. Child-parent psychotherapy: a developmental approach to mental health treatment in infancy and early childhood. In: Zeanah C, editor. Handbook of infant mental health. 3rd Edition. New York: Guilford Press; 2009. p. 439–49 Chapter 27.

63. Lieberman AF, Silverman R, Pawl JH. Infant-parent psychotherapy: core concepts and current approaches. In: Zeanah C, editor. Handbook of infant mental health. 2nd edition. New York: Guilford Press; 2000. p. 472–84.

Training Child Psychiatrists in Family-Based Integrated Care

Michelle L. Rickerby, MD[a],*, Thomas A. Roesler, MD[b]

KEYWORDS

- Family systems • Family therapy • Family-based treatment • Integrated care
- Patient-centered care • Patient- and family-centered care • Child psychiatry training

KEY POINTS

- Evidence supports that family-based assessment and intervention are essential skills for child psychiatrists.
- Family-based training can occur in child psychiatry residency in a way that complements other aspects of training and equips trainees for a broad range of real-world practice settings.
- The heuristic model of family-based integrated care (FBIC) guides case formulation in the context of family beliefs and relationships in support of productive joining with families and optimal integration of treatment across illnesses and levels of care.
- The application of the FBIC model is effective in the management of several broadly experienced challenges that occur in child psychiatry practice. Some of these challenges include family conflict over treatment recommendations, parental avoidance of limit setting, and family relationships impaired by destructive affect and disconnection.
- Trainees exposed to this FBIC training report positive impact from the training in their ongoing professional activities in a variety of settings.

OVERVIEW

This issue of *Child and Adolescent Psychiatric Clinics of North America* makes the case that child psychiatrists, to have an ongoing and significant impact on the children they treat, must include family context considerations in all aspects of practice. Few fellowship training programs adequately prepare trainees to think and respond systemically. Child Psychiatry as a field has been challenged to integrate family therapy

Drs M.L. Rickerby and T.A. Roesler have no disclosures.
[a] The Hasbro Children's Partial Hospital Program, 593 Eddy Street, Providence, RI 02906, USA;
[b] Psychiatry and Behavioral Medicine Unit, Seattle Children's Hospital, University of Washington School of Medicine, 4800 Sandpoint Way Northeast, Seattle, WA 98105, USA
* Corresponding author.
E-mail address: MRickerby@Lifespan.org

Abbreviations	
ADHD	Attention-deficit hyperactivity disorder
CBT	Cognitive-behavioral therapy
HCPHP	Hasbro Children's Partial Hospital Program
DBT	Dialectical-behavior therapy
FBIC	Family-based integrated care

comfortably from the outset. Ehrlich described this in a 1972 paper. "There appears to be an uneasiness in finding a place for family therapy in child psychiatry."[1] He continued, "It is our impression that family interviewing is considered a special and difficult procedure to be undertaken only by those with particular interest, skill, or experience."[1] At the time, tension centered on the conceptual shift away from psychoanalytically oriented psychotherapy. There has been a trend toward substantially less overall psychotherapy training in both General and Child Psychiatry Residency Training programs.[2–7] Pressures contributing to this trend include the rapidly growing volume of neurodevelopmental, genetic, epigenetic, and pharmacologic information; the relative shortage of child psychiatrists; and the practice of psychotherapy by a range of other disciplines.[8] Upcoming shifts toward recently modified core competencies in child psychiatry training and the transition to Diagnostic and Statistical Manual of Mental Disorders, Fifth Edition, offer an opportunity to reorganize training in this area.[9–16]

Despite this trend, there is growing evidence supporting the critical impact of the family on children's mental health.[8,17–22] This impact is seen in research involving epigenetics, the effects of toxic stress and parental mental illness, and interventions involving family-based treatment. Psychosocially oriented evidence-based treatments often focus on the details of the illness or symptoms without an eye to context. However, as addressed in other articles in this issue, these interventions function better when they incorporate family systems components.

THE TRAINING MODEL: HOW TRAINEES ARE EXPOSED TO FAMILY SYSTEMS THINKING

We developed the Family Therapy Training program for the Child Psychiatry and Triple Board Residency Programs of The Alpert School of Medicine of Brown University during a 15-year period between 1998 and 2013 (Other contributors to the development of the training program include Charles Malone, MD [1998–2002]; Robert Pazulinec, PhD [2001–2009]; and David McConville PhD [2010–present]). The program was part of a comprehensive training experience that included exposure to a variety of psychotherapeutic interventions, psychopharmacologic treatments, and experience in several practice settings. It was our task and our desire to develop a training experience that complemented what colleagues were teaching the trainees. We set out to add family systems thinking to the world view our trainees were exposed to as they readied themselves to practice child psychiatry. Other programs have reported on the productive use of "family evaluation clinics"[3] and an "experiential interdisciplinary course,"[2] but a survey of 7 US child psychiatry training programs in 2011 found that, although fellows considered exposure to family intervention valuable, most had not seen more than 1 outpatient family with supervision during their training.[6]

The training model incorporates the following:

- Ten hours of didactics on family therapy concepts
- One year experience in a family therapy training clinic
- Two years of group supervision

- Four hours of didactics on couples' therapy
- Elective exposure to individual supervision with a family therapy supervisor

This schedule approximates 140 to 160 hours of direct instruction during 2 years. There are 5 child psychiatry fellows and 3 Triple Board residents per year in each year of the 2-year training. Group supervision is divided by training year: the first year fellows combine with fourth year Triple Board residents and second year fellows with fifth year Triple Board residents. Thus, cohorts are 8 trainees per year.

The 10 hours of teaching on family therapy concepts occurs in 3 workshop sessions in July-August of the academic year for the cohort entering their first year of child psychiatry fellowship and fourth year of Triple Board residency. The faculty agreed that early training in family concepts was a necessary part of the tool kit every child psychiatrist in training needs as he or she begins fellowship.

INTRODUCTORY SEMINARS

Major topic areas in these first seminars include Genograms; Joining Strategies; Pattern Identification in Family Systems; and Interventive Interviewing techniques.[23] Sessions are team taught by us and a staff psychologist who runs the family therapy training clinic. Use of videotaped examples of family therapy sessions, demonstration interviews, and role plays are incorporated into these sessions.

By creating genograms, trainees make a commitment to understanding the child in a family context. Joining skill building focuses on the challenge of connecting simultaneously with multiple family members in a developmentally appropriate way. In role plays and discussions about the joining process, residents learn how to gain an understanding of family belief systems in a manner that is experienced as supportive by the family. Practice with pattern identification in families serves to develop a working vocabulary of relationally focused terms and to establish comfort for the trainee in observing painful or otherwise challenging relationship patterns. The introduction to interventive interviewing techniques gives a preview for the trainees to the power of language as therapists help families find new patterns of thinking, feeling, and behaving. Residents are encouraged to shift from a default linear viewpoint of causation to a circular and reflexive vision. This is the most challenging piece of the introductory curriculum.

COGNITIVE AND AFFECTIVE/SPATIAL DIMENSIONS IN FAMILY SYSTEMS THERAPY

It is in this introduction to family systems therapy that we first use "the graph." (**Fig. 1**) While recognizing there are many dimensions that describe the quality of life in families, if students are encouraged to pay attention to a cognitive dimension (eg, the presence of ongoing beliefs either shared or idiosyncratic to 1 family member) and an affective/spatial dimension (eg, relationships between family members that generate emotional states and affect the ability to problem solve), then the students have a way to evaluate where the child and family is at the start of treatment and at any time along the course of treatment. A significant portion of this article is dedicated to demonstrating how these concepts translate into treatment strategies.

The family therapy training clinic in which residents participate during the first year of this 2-year curriculum is supervised by an outpatient staff psychologist. All residents engage in 1 to 2 hours per week of family therapy with direct supervision from the psychology attending during at least half of each session. Residents are encouraged to practice family formulation and joining and to be focused on "where the family is" with beliefs and relationships. Trainees typically rely more on the

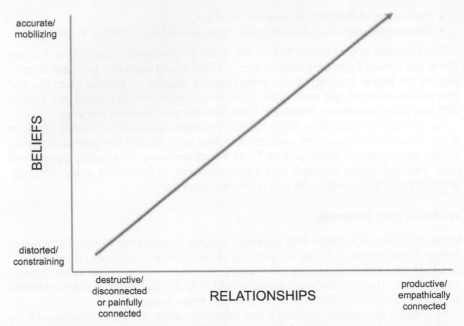

Fig. 1. Family-based integrated care graph.

experienced faculty member in the beginning as they practice shifting from linear interviewing to systems theory–directed observation and interviewing. Sessions are videotaped with family consent. In addition to direct supervision, further discussion occurs before or after sessions as well as in the context of group supervision during which time videotape is reviewed in detail.

Group supervision during the first and second year of the curriculum involves trainees taking turns sharing case material from families they are actively treating. Although most commonly cases are from their outpatient panels, they are encouraged to bring cases that they are treating in any context for support around family-based treatment. It is not unusual that trainees may bring for supervision a patient they initially began treating with individual therapy but have realized that further family involvement is essential. A common tool in the group supervision setting is the use of role playing the same moment seen on video, in real time, with the group brainstorming productive questions to highlight the therapeutic message that will broaden the family's perspective. There is repeated emphasis on using the FBIC model, and referring to the graph, to center the trainees' formulation as they enter each session and to use this as an anchor to preplan a set of circular and reflexive questions that support family movement toward mobilizing beliefs and empathic connections.

The second year of group supervision has the same structure as the first. During the second year, residents are much more comfortable with seeing family context as foreground with respect to symptoms. With the second year, trainee discussion shifts toward more complex strategizing to support family movement away from beliefs that are constraining or inaccurate and toward more empathic and growth-promoting relationships. Rather than practicing circular and reflexive questions that help clarify the relationship and belief status quo as was the case in the first year, the emphasis is on creating momentum for family-based shifts from observed patterns to more functional ones. The other conceptual leap that residents at this level of training embrace is the application of family systems concepts to the bigger picture of coordination of care for patients as well as to their own functioning in systems of care in the hospital system. Couples' therapy didactic sessions are interwoven in the second year of group supervision sessions.

THE TRAINING MODEL: WHAT TRAINEES NEED TO LEARN
Hasbro Children's Partial Hospital Program

Most trainees receiving instruction in family systems also do clinical rotations on the Hasbro Children's Partial Hospital Program (HCPHP) whereby they have an opportunity to observe and participate in FBIC being delivered to children and teens with complex pediatric illness.[24] This hospital program, also developed by us, provides a living laboratory where trainees can see the concepts taught in seminars and supervision in action with children and their families receiving an intense intervention for long-standing medical and psychiatric issues.

It is often while working on the HCPHP that trainees come to appreciate that FBIC is not simply involving the family in a child's treatment plan. It is not just using family therapy as a treatment modality. It is a meta viewpoint from which every treatment decision is made, taking into consideration that family relationships and family beliefs about the illness together constitute the most powerful force in illness management and recovery.[25–27] Integrated care is more than jointly conceptualizing physical and psychological issues. Integration in this model involves the coordination of all modalities of care through communication across providers and the provision of a common message about illness and treatment to patients and families.

Symptoms in Family-Based Cognitive Relational Context

The graph is a constant reminder to trainees that symptoms must be placed in a family-based cognitive, relational context. Although we have used the graph as a teaching tool with naive groups as an introduction to family systems thinking, as we did in the first weeks of fellowship training, our trainees come to appreciate complexity in family organization by coming back to the graph over and over, with new understanding as they see more families in treatment.

Trainees come to see that the expression of the symptom or presenting problem, which is not even included on the graph, is deeply affected by where a family is plotted on the 2 dimensions.

They come to see that a focus on symptoms/illness outside of the multidimensional context represented by the graph has the potential to grant the illness more power over the patient and family's life rather than less. An example of this common to child psychiatric practice is the process of decision making around suicidality and level of care. There are situations in which context dictates that, even when suicidality is intense, the most therapeutic option is for a patient to remain home surrounded by family support. Meanwhile, other situations in which suicidality is less intense but family relationships are less nurturing necessitates an inpatient level of care.

Subjectivity in Observations

There is occasional criticism that a therapist is being judgmental by plotting observed beliefs or relationships; that rating, for example, a certain belief as falling somewhere along a continuum between "distorted/constraining versus accurate/mobilizing." There is an element of judgment involved. However, when a family is asked, "is this belief you just expressed more likely to keep things from getting better or to help you move in new directions," most families agree with the therapist's judgment.

We feel safe to say, and our trainees come to believe this as well, that whatever illness that is causing pain and distress, movement toward accurate illness beliefs and empathic, productive relationships diminish pain and distress for the patient.

Dynamic Beliefs and Relationships

Beliefs and relationships have lives of their own. But they are not static. They respond to life circumstances, new evidence, and even therapeutic interventions. They shift, and so the plotting of an individual or shared belief can change, sometimes in front of our eyes, and the therapist must be constantly able to shift his or her evaluation of what is happening as this is taking place.

We teach trainees to be on the look out for contradictory beliefs within the same family or even within one individual. Such beliefs are not likely to provide aid in problem solving. Likewise, we pay special attention to relationship constellations that push for less versus more empathy. As a trainee comes to know a family better, multiple points can be plotted for beliefs in any given family as is the case for recognizing multiple relationships with varying characteristics.

Evaluating families asking for help for their child in this way has several advantages that become apparent with experience. It inherently generates a feeling in families that someone is listening to them. It allows for a richer discussion between disciplines and smoother transitions across levels of care. It provides a sense of reassurance for both treatment providers and those receiving treatment that we know where we are at any given time in treatment. Taken together, these features result in improved morale, both for the treatment team and for the family. It allows our trainee to step back from the distorted thinking and painful relationships in the therapy room and say, "well at least I know where we are and where we need to go," which can be an incredibly freeing experience.

Understanding where a family is on the graph, understanding the context on at least two dimensions in which symptoms are being expressed, is especially important in one all too common experience in child psychiatry; this is the ability to avoid having patients with a clearly diagnosed illness be discharged with "better controlled symptoms" while little is understood about the context they are returning to at home. These children all too often have exacerbations of symptoms resulting in readmission to the hospital.

Advantages of Family-Based Model to Psychiatrist-Trainee

For trainees, in particular, the FBIC model can help combat an expectable sense of helplessness as well as the tendency to overfocus on symptoms and illness categories rather than on the patient who has the illness. The meta view of "knowing where the family is," even if it is a troubled, painful place, is a relief as it naturally implies a path forward. In addition, although trainees may often feel daunted by the power of any particular illness entity, they can shift to feeling empowered with the understanding that regardless of the severity of the illness they can intervene in the family system in a manner that offers relief while the patient and family live with the illness.

The child fellow and Triple Board trainees trained in this program should be able to use their skills and new way of thinking across the entirety of their child psychiatry practice. We believe the exposure to the FBIC model provides a core belief system to guide treatment decisions across schools of psychotherapy and levels of care. It offers a scaffolding to which they can affix a broad range of interventions that they are adding to their tool kit including evidence-based psychopharmacology and manualized models of cognitive-behavioral therapy (CBT) and dialectical-behavior therapy (DBT). Any of these specific interventions can be mapped onto the patient and family treatment trajectory as guided by the graph. When anchored to the real context, trainees have a greater sense of competence in making each decision in a therapeutic way across a trajectory of treatment.

By the beginning of the second year of training, our students are ready to assess and make interventions in situations that cause many experienced clinicians to feel challenged and sometimes defeated. We are seeing repeated scenarios such as the ones described here. The process we follow in walking them through the challenging situations is discussed further.

THE TRAINING MODEL: CLINICAL APPLICATIONS
Family Conflict About Treatment Recommendations

CASE VIGNETTE

A 9-year-old boy presents for treatment of long-standing hyperactive and impulsive behavior at home and school. He has been diagnosed with attention-deficit hyperactivity disorder (ADHD) in past evaluations and has reportedly had little success to date with either stimulant trials or therapy focused on parental behavior management. In the interview, Mom is focused on finding the right medication, whereas Dad is hopeless that anything will help his out of control son.

The belief axis
In this family, both parents present with different strong beliefs that leave them feeling disempowered in different ways. Mom's overfocus on medication as the complete solution leaves her missing the bigger picture that for children with ADHD the structure and messages provided by their environment are critical to supporting their growth in self-control. Dad's expressed hopelessness reflects his belief that neither his son nor he has any ability to make choices that might lead to control of these overwhelming symptoms. Both parents' beliefs likely predispose them to offer messages to their son that convey both he and they are helpless in the face of symptoms, likely leaving him demoralized and disempowered as well. This belief context is one that provides fertile ground for oppositional behavior patterns and depressive symptoms, common comorbidities with ADHD, to take root and flourish.

The relationship axis
The relationship between the parents in this scenario is characterized by distance and disagreement. This situation likely has led to conflict between them and mixed messages from them to their son. It is also likely that each parent's relationship with their son is characterized by distance and distress, potentially leading him to feel blamed for his symptoms being out of control, promoting anger and further acting out on his part, thereby leading to symptom magnification rather than reduction.

FBIC intervention
The goal in this situation is to generate a shift toward a broader family view of factors that influence the child's behavior, higher joining and lower conflict between parents, and empathic clear messages about taking responsibility from parents to child.

Circular questions that offer a frame to expand beliefs include the following:

- Recently, when the medication for his ADHD was not working, how much of his outbursts do you believe he can control versus not control?

- What percentage of his behavior being under good control feels like it comes from medication versus his own efforts versus your coaching him in calming down?
- As we work together to identify the right medication to help with the part of the ADHD that is out of all of your control, what message do you want your son to get about what you can do to help him with this challenge? What message do you want him to get about what he can do to help?
- Circular questions aimed at addressing distant and unempathic relationships include "When your son's behavior is most out of control, what is the saddest part for him?"
- Mom (or Dad), what does your husband (or wife) most misunderstand about what is hardest for you in parenting your son?
- When the household is under pressure given how out of control things have felt, would your son say it pulls you two closer together to be a team managing things or pushes you apart because of frustration?

This version of interventive interviewing allows the clinician to obtain more detailed information about family beliefs and relationships and introduce expanded beliefs and bridges between family members in an immediately productive way.

The Family Protection Fallacy

CASE VIGNETTE

Married parents present to the crisis clinic with their 12-year-old son who has recently been refusing to attend school. He has been irritable and shut down at home. Parents feel helpless and afraid and note "but he has always been such a good student." Mom was recently diagnosed with breast cancer for which she is to begin treatment next week.

The belief axis
At first glance it seems that the parents in this situation may not believe that their son's behavior is connected to the bigger picture of family distress. It is also likely that they believe that shielding him from discussion about Mom's cancer will make it easier for him. Common reasons for children to be shut down in this situation may include a belief that "talking won't make anything better" and that if they share their upset "it will just make my parents more upset and they're already going through a lot."

The relationship axis
Family member's attempts to shield each other from pain by not talking about upsetting topics can lead to more distance between people, which magnifies pain rather than reduces it. Families with strongly empathic connections at baseline are at risk of falling into this family protection fallacy. It is also likely that in this scenario, parent's sensitivity to their son's upset about his mother's condition, although perhaps not discussed, is leading them to back off on usual limits and expectations that would support his school attendance. They might note, "we know he is dealing with so much already."

FBIC intervention
In this scenario, shifting the family's belief about shielding each other from pain by not discussing it to the empowered stance that being together in pain diminishes its destructive force is paramount.

Examples of questions focused on supporting this belief shift include the following:

- What is your Dad worried would happen if he were able to let you know just how upset he is about your mom's cancer diagnosis?
- If your son told you his greatest fear about your cancer what is he worried might happen?

A question focused on shifting relationships to maximize empathy and closeness in such a situation includes multiple versions of the following:

- A large stress like adjusting to a cancer diagnosis can pull families together, push them apart, or both. What would your son/husband/wife/mother/father say is happening with your family?

Embedded within these questions is a normalizing framework that offers a message of respecting the care family members have for each other while encouraging them to rely on that strength most productively in this crisis.

Family Impairment Related to Destructive Affect: Blame

CASE VIGNETTE

Married parents bring their 13-year-old daughter for an outpatient evaluation after catching her smoking marijuana. The father is frequently absent from home because of a demanding schedule of work-related travel. The mother blames his lack of presence in the home for his daughter's behavior. Dad openly blames Mom for not being a firm limit setter.

The belief axis

Both parents in this situation are conveying a belief that they are not part of the problem and thereby cannot be a part of the solution. This blame deadlock is thereby profoundly disempowering as it leaves each feeling helpless. Any message they may attempt to give their daughter about her taking responsibility for her behavior is meaningless in this culture of blame. Her belief likely will be that everyone else is to blame except her.

The relationship axis

Blame creates smoke that prevents family members from addressing their own guilt and shame, which most often is what interferes with their ability to take responsibility for their part. Without taking responsibility mobilization is not possible, which can then magnify blame cycles. This dynamic necessarily distances family members from each other, leaving them alone and defensive rather than connected and able to address their vulnerabilities.

FBIC intervention

In this common scenario, conversation that supports each family member shifting from blaming others to taking responsibility for his or her own contribution to the crisis at hand is the key. That belief shift can lead to stronger parent joining and clearer messages to children. Such a shift can allow family members to feel better about themselves and each other, generating healthier relationships.

Two versions of a core question aimed at supporting this belief and relationship shift are as follows:

- "As much as you blame your husband's lack of availability for your daughter's self-destructive behavior, what is the piece you are most faulting yourself for?"

- "As much as your husband blames your softness with limits for your daughter's self-destructive behavior, what is he most beating himself up for in this situation?"

Although both questions offer a frame to support each person sharing their vulnerability in an effort to become more empowered, the latter delivers more relationship impact by creating a potential bridge between parents while the same theme is explored.

Other examples that bridge to the daughter as well are the following:

- "Does your daughter struggle more with anger at others because she blames them for her current crisis, or more with anger at herself over the situation?"
- "What is the saddest part for your daughter as she sits here and hears the two of you blame each other for her self-destructive behavior?"

The use of questions that support frame shifting as well as bridging between family members is a powerful tool for guiding families out of the nonproductive loop of blame.

Family Impairment Related to Destructive Affect: Anger

> **CASE VIGNETTE**
>
> *Recently divorced parents of a 16-year-old girl admitted inpatient after a potentially lethal suicide attempt via acetaminophen (Tylenol) overdose present for a family meeting in the inpatient psychiatric unit. The parents expression of intense anger toward each other leaves their daughter in tears and resistant to participating in the discussion.*

The belief axis

In situations of unmitigated rage between parents, there is often either tunnel vision or complete blindness limiting their ability to believe that their anger is destructive to their children. The above-mentioned situation also likely has a good dose of counterproductive blame beliefs mixed in as well. This level of destructive anger most often leaves children with the belief that their parents do not care about them.

The relationship axis

Anger pushes other people away. Family members blinded by rage often get further and further apart at times when a sense of connection is desperately needed. Although this intensity of animosity can often lead clinicians to reflexively pull back, leaning in to the underlying issues is an opportunity to bridge family members. Often, there is an underlying fear of loss or actual loss that fuels this intensity of anger.

FBIC intervention

In a family blinded and disempowered by rage, the clinician's goal is to support heightened awareness around the belief that parental animosity and hatred is toxic for children. In addition, the goal is to bring out the underlying loss and sadness that provide fuel for the anger.

Questions aimed at heightening parents' awareness around the impact of their anger on their children include the following:

- "What is the saddest part for your daughter when she sees the two of you ripping into each other the way that you are?"
- "Does your daughter become more angry or sad when she hears the two of you fighting like this?"

The assumption of the daughter's sadness is not in question; rather it is embedded in the question, which serves to join with her while you are directing the question toward the parents.

Questions aimed at addressing the underlying issues limiting connection between family members include the following:

- "As pissed off as you are right now at your ex-wife, what is the part that you are feeling saddest about for your family at this moment?"
- "If the anger between you wasn't so intense how might you be working together right now to support your daughter after her suicide attempt?"

It is critical that discussions in such circumstances acknowledge the real presence and impact of destructive anger and are aimed at joining with all family members around the underlying pain and sadness. In such circumstances, the therapist has a line of vision that the family does not.

Stress-Related Tunnel Vision

CASE VIGNETTE

A 16-year-old boy recently diagnosed with type I diabetes presents to the crisis clinic with his mother because of explosive behavior and frequent violation of his curfew. His elevated blood sugars have almost led to medical admission in recent weeks. The teenager reports that "when I'm home my mother is constantly making me check my blood sugar...she is out of control!" This is a single parent household.

The belief axis
It is common in the setting of medical illness like diabetes for parents to have catastrophic thinking about their teenager managing the illness. For example, this Mom might say, "If I let him out of my sight I worry he might die." Meanwhile, teen bravado commonly colors beliefs toward risky denial. This teen might state, "I don't need to check my blood sugar, I can tell what it is by how I feel." A common pattern in families is that the overreactive beliefs of one member can magnify the underreactive beliefs of another.

The relationship axis
Variations in stress responsiveness or lack of understanding each other's perspectives can foster conflict and disconnection in situations in which teamwork is essential. It is common in such scenarios for the normal privacy of teenagers to become magnified into secrecy, which creates distance in relationships, thus removing the protectiveness that is essential in parent-child relationships.

FBIC intervention
The goal here is to generate dialogue that promotes awareness about how extremes of beliefs can limit mobilization. In addition, the focus is on discussion of the inadvertent distance that differential coping with crisis can generate.

The following are examples of questions aimed at less constraining and more realistic beliefs:

- "For some people understanding how serious diabetes can be can be mobilizing and lead to action while for others it can be overwhelming to a point that they can become paralyzed. Sometimes it can be both. What would your son/mother say is happening for you?"

- "As much as your mother worries how you handle your diabetes when you are out on your own, what part does she trust you most with?"
- "As much as your son can tend to blow off caring for his diabetes, and sometimes pretend like he doesn't have it, what part scares him the most?"

Discussion aimed at relationship valence in this situation might include questions such as the following:

- "Does the fact that your son knows how scared you are about him dying from his diabetes make it more or less likely that he is comfortable asking for your help with it day to day?"
- "If I asked your mother whether the stress of diabetes was more pulling you two together or pushing you apart or both, what would she say?"

Even when people seem to have extreme beliefs, they can often appreciate or understand a conflicting belief in someone with whom they are close. Making room for this in discussions with families can allow them to feel more connected even when some disagreement persists.

THE TRAINING MODEL: EVALUATING THE LONG-TERM OUTCOME

The Brown Family Therapy Training Program functioned consistently from 1998 to 2013. In preparation for this publication, we wanted to learn the effect the training had on the trainees now out in the real world. To accomplish this, we collaborated with The Brown University Child Psychiatry and Triple Board Residency Training Director in conducting a survey distributed via e-mail in June 2014. The survey was distributed to N = 126 graduates of the Brown Child Psychiatry and Triple Board Residency Programs. Contact information was not available for a small proportion of trainees (N = 10) who were not included in the survey. Of those surveyed, there was a 91% response rate (N = 115) (**Table 1**).

Given the high response rate and acceptable distribution, the data are considered to be a valid representation of opinions for graduates of the Brown Training Program during this period.

The respondents represent a broad range of practice settings and modalities of practice (**Tables 2** and **3**).

Respondent practicing with a range of treatment modalities and roles is typical in current child psychiatric practice.

Questions about the utility of their family therapy training yielded consistently high ratings across respondents (**Table 4**).

Most of those who responded to the training survey considered their family therapy training to be useful in their professional life. This data serves to support the idea that FBIC training can occur in child psychiatry residency in a way that complements other aspects of training and equips trainees for a broad range of real-world practice settings.

Table 1	
Respondents to the Brown 2014 Training Impact Survey	
Response Rate	91% (N = 115)
Child Psychiatry Residency Graduates	57% (N = 66)
Triple Board Residency Graduates	43% (N = 39)

Table 2
Practice settings of survey respondents

Full-time practice	67.9%
Academic affiliation	37.9%
Hospital based	43.2%
Community based	20.7%
Private practice	25.9%
Inpatient	27.6%
Outpatient	50%
Partial programs	15.5%

Table 3
Practice modalities of survey respondents

Pharmacologic treatment	91.4%
Individual therapy	67.2%
Family therapy	60.3%
Group therapy	13.8%
Pediatric consultation	34.5%
School consultation	20.7%
Administration	44.8%
Teaching	65.5%
Research	29.3%

Table 4
Utility of family systems training to current practice

Experience/Skill	Somewhat Useful (%)	Very Useful (%)	Composite Usefulness (%)
Didactics	20	79	99
Group supervision	25	68	93
Individual supervision	15	85	100
Couples' therapy Didactics/supervision	57	34	91
Joining	27	69	96
Assessment	14	86	100
Circular questioning	25	72	97
Family therapy as primary modality	40	56	96

SUMMARY

Despite the trend toward a decreased emphasis on family therapy training in child psychiatry during the past 2 decades, evidence from a small retrospective survey about a model program at Brown University during the same period demonstrates that training in family assessment and intervention can be integrated into residency and provide skills that are considered highly useful across postgraduate practice settings. Although the lack of a sample of similar data across training programs nationally prevents determination of whether trainees exposed to less robust family-based training feel ill-equipped in practice, the near unanimity of positive response is notable.[1,2,18,23]

The heuristic model of FBIC has the potential to provide a scaffold from which to construct an updated curriculum for child psychiatry residents in training that meets modern challenges. It demonstrates the flexibility to provide a family-based vision that can be incorporated across modalities and levels of care. In addition, the FBIC model may be useful across mental health disciplines as a training paradigm on which a broad range of evidence-based models of intervention can be graphed. Treatment ranging from individually delivered CBT or DBT to parent training to pharmacotherapy all have a place within this broader vision. Knowing where the family is on the FBIC graph can help organize joining, cross-discipline communication, and level-of-care decisions in a manner that may maximize family mobilization and thereby support optimal patient outcomes.

REFERENCES

1. Ehrlich FM. Family therapy training and child psychiatry. J Am Acad Child Psychiatry 1973;12(3):461–72.
2. Carrey N, Costanzo L, Sexton A, et al. The Dalhousie Family Therapy Training Program: Our 6 Year Experience. Can Child Adolesc Psychiatr Rev 2004;13(4): 114–8.
3. Celano M, Croft S, Morrissey-Kane E. Family evaluation clinic: training psychiatrists to think systemically. Acad Psychiatry 2002;26(1):17–25.
4. Heru A, Keitner G, Glick I. Family therapy: the neglected core competence. Acad Psychiatry 2012;36(6):433–5.
5. Kovach JG, Dubin WR, Combs CJ. Psychotherapy training: resident's perceptions and experiences. Acad Psychiatry 2014. [Epub ahead of print].
6. Rait DS. Family therapy training in child and adolescent psychiatry fellowship programs. Acad Psychiatry 2012;36(6):448–51.
7. Sexson SB. Overview of training in the twenty-first century. Child Adolesc Psychiatr Clin N Am 2007;16(1):1–16.
8. Patterson J, Vakili S. Relationships, environment, and the brain: how emerging research is changing what we know about the impact of families on human development. Fam Process 2014;53(1):22–32.
9. Chrisman AK, Enderlin HT, Landry KL, et al. Teaching evidence-based medicine pediatric psychopharmacology: integrating psychopharmacologic treatment into the broad spectrum of care. Child Adolesc Psychiatr Clin N Am 2007;16(1): 165–81.
10. Dingle AD. The DSM-5: an opportunity to affirm "the whole child" concept in child and adolescent psychiatric residency training. Acad Psychiatry 2014;38(1):64–6.
11. Havighurst SS, Downey L. Clinical reasoning for child and adolescent mental health practitioners: the mindful formulation. Clin Child Psychol Psychiatry 2009;14(2):251–71.

12. Josephson AM. Reinventing family therapy: teaching family intervention as a new treatment modality. Acad Psychiatry 2008;32(5):405–13.
13. Josephson AM. Family intervention as a developmental psychodynamic psychotherapy. Child Adolesc Psychiatr Clin N Am 2013;22(2):241–60.
14. McGinty KL. Training child and adolescent psychiatrists for systems of care. Psychiatr Serv 2003;54(1):29–30.
15. McGinty KL, Larson JJ, Hodas G, et al. Teaching patient centered care and systems-based practice in child and adolescent psychiatry. Acad Psychiatry 2012;36(6):468–72.
16. Scholl I, Jordis MZ, Harter M, et al. An integrative model of patient-centeredness - a systematic review and concept analysis. PLos One 2014;9(9):e107828.
17. Kaslow NJ, Broth MR, Smith CO, et al. Family based interventions for child and adolescent disorders. J Marital Fam Ther 2012;38(91):82–100.
18. Retzlaff R, Von Sydow K, Behar S, et al. The efficacy of systemic therapy for internalizing and other disorders of childhood and adolescence: a systematic review of 38 randomized controlled trials. Fam Process 2014;32(4):619–52.
19. Scott S. Parenting quality and children's mental health: biological mechanisms and psychological interventions. Curr Opin Psychiatry 2012;25(4):301–6.
20. Siegenthaler E, Munder T, Egger M. Effect of preventive interventions in mentally ill parents on the mental health of the offspring: systematic review and meta-analysis. J Am Acad Child Adolesc Psychiatry 2012;51(1):8–17.
21. Wamboldt MZ, Wamboldt FS. Role of the family in the onset and outcome of childhood disorders: selected research findings. J Am Acad Child Adolesc Psychiatry 2000;39(10):1212–9.
22. Von Sydow K, Retzlaff R, Behar S, et al. The efficacy of systemic therapy for childhood and adolescent externalizing disorders: a systematic review of 47 randomized controlled trials. Fam Process 2013;52(4):576–618.
23. Thomm K. Interventive interviewing: Part III. Intending to ask lineal, circular, strategic, or reflexive questions. Fam Process 1988;27:1–15.
24. Roesler TA, Rickerby ML, Nassau JH, et al. Treating a high risk population: a collaboration of child psychiatry and pediatrics. Med Health R I 2002;85(9):265–8.
25. DiMatteo MR. Variations in patients' adherence to medical recommendations: a quantitative review of 50 years of research. Med Care 2004;42(3):200–9.
26. DiMatteo MR, Haskard KB, Williams SL. Health beliefs, disease severity, and patient adherence: a meta-analysis. Med Care 2007;45(6):521–8.
27. Vermeire E, Hearnshaw H, Van Royen P, et al. Patient adherence to treatment: three decades of research. a comprehensive review. J Clin Pharm Ther 2001;26(5):331–42.

Family-Based Interventions for Childhood Mood Disorders

Andrea S. Young, PhD[a], Mary A. Fristad, PhD, ABPP[a,b,*]

KEYWORDS

- Bipolar spectrum disorder • Depressive spectrum disorders • Children
- Adolescents • Psychosis • Psychotherapy • Evidence-based treatment
- Family-based treatment

KEY POINTS

- Family psychoeducation (FPE) plus skill building is the only psychotherapy identified as probably efficacious for childhood bipolar spectrum disorders (BPSDs), although none have been identified as well established.
- Cognitive behavioral therapy (CBT) is considered well established for childhood depressive spectrum disorders (DSDs).
- Few studies examine psychotherapy for young children in randomized controlled trials (RCTs).
- Family-based therapy has repeatedly demonstrated greater symptom improvement than treatment as usual among children with mood disorders in RCTs.
- Common components of efficacious family-based therapies include psychoeducation; problem-solving, communication, and social skills building; as well as cognitive reframing.
- The benefits of family-based therapy over individual therapy for childhood depression remain unclear.

OVERVIEW OF CHILDHOOD MOOD DISORDERS

Mood disorders (bipolar spectrum disorder [BPSD] and depressive spectrum disorder [DSD]) are debilitating psychiatric problems that affect both youth and adults. These disorders are associated with impaired functioning in relationships with family and

Disclosures: None (A.S. Young); Dr M.A. Fristad receives royalties from Guilford Press, American Psychiatric Press, and Child & Family Psychological Services, Inc.
[a] Department of Psychiatry and Behavioral Health, The Ohio State University, 1670 Upham Drive, Suite 460, Columbus, OH 43210, USA; [b] Departments of Psychology and Nutrition, The Ohio State University, 1670 Upham Drive, Suite 460, Columbus, OH 43210, USA
* Corresponding author. Department of Psychiatry and Behavioral Health, The Ohio State University, 1670 Upham Drive, Suite 460, Columbus, OH 43210.
E-mail address: mary.fristad@osumc.edu

Child Adolesc Psychiatric Clin N Am 24 (2015) 517–534
http://dx.doi.org/10.1016/j.chc.2015.02.008
1056-4993/15/$ – see front matter © 2015 Elsevier Inc. All rights reserved.

childpsych.theclinics.com

Abbreviations

ABFT	Attachment-Based Family Therapy
ADHD	Attention-deficit/hyperactivity disorder
BD-I	Bipolar I disorder
BD-II	Bipolar II disorder
BPSD	Bipolar spectrum disorder
CBT	Cognitive behavioral therapy
CFF-CBT	Child- and family-focused CBT
DBT	Dialectical behavior therapy
DSM	*Diagnostic and Statistical Manual of Mental Disorders*
DSD	Depressive spectrum disorder
FBPs	Family-based psychotherapies
FFT-A	Family-Focused Treatment for Adolescents
FFT-HR	Family-Focused Therapy-High Risk
FIPP	Focused Individual Psychodynamic Psychotherapy
FPE	Family psychoeducation
IF-PEP	Individual-Family Psychoeducational Psychotherapy
MDD	Major depressive disorder
MF-PEP	Multi-Family Psychoeducational Psychotherapy
PCIT	Parent-Child Interaction Therapy
PCIT-ED	Parent-Child Interaction Therapy-Emotion Development
RCTs	Randomized controlled trials
SIFT	Systems Integrative Family Therapy
SSRI	Selective serotonin reuptake inhibitor
TAU	Treatment as usual
WLC	Wait list control

peers, cognitive abilities, and performance at work and school. Onset of mood disorders in childhood can lead to long-term impairment and increased risk of mood symptoms in adulthood.[1,2]

PREVALENCE, PRESENTATION, AND COMORBIDITIES

Despite considerable debate regarding whether children can truly have a BPSD, substantial evidence now supports its presentation in youth.[2] Childhood BPSD has an estimated prevalence rate of 1.8%, and the prevalence in adolescents is 2.7%.[3] Prevalence of DSD is higher, with estimated rates of 2.8% in childhood and 5.7% in adolescence.[4]

Children with mood disorders often have a complex constellation of symptoms and are at high risk for future psychiatric problems. Childhood-onset major depressive disorder (MDD) is associated with greater risk for suicide, substance abuse, behavioral problems, and increased risk for having a DSD in adolescence and adulthood.[1,5] Childhood-onset MDD is associated with greater risk for later BPSD than is adult-onset MDD[6]; 20% to 40% of youth with MDD will have a BPSD later in life.[5]

Symptom presentation of MDD in youth is similar to that in adults in many ways; however, children are less likely to experience hypersomnia, decreased appetite, and delusions compared to adults.[6] While some youth do have a classic BD presentation (ie, sustained periods of irritable or elated mood lasting for days at a time), children with BPSD are more likely to exhibit rapid cycling, or shorter periods of extreme irritable or elated mood[7] and are at high risk for relapse after remission.[2,7] Kowatch and colleagues[8] found that estimated rates of manic symptoms in youth with BPSD are fairly similar across childhood BPSD studies, with the most common symptoms being increased energy, distractibility, pressured speech, and irritability. Among children with subsyndromal bipolar disorder (bipolar disorder not otherwise specified [BD-NOS] in *Diagnostic and Statistical Manual of Mental Disorders* [Fourth Edition] [DSM-IV][9] or other specified bipolar and related disorder in DSM-V[10]), about one-third meet the criteria for bipolar I disorder (BD-I) or bipolar II disorder (BD-II) within 2 to 4 years.[11]

Most children with mood disorders have comorbid diagnoses. Common comorbidities for BPSD and DSD include attention-deficit/hyperactivity disorder (ADHD), disruptive behavior, anxiety, and (in adolescents) substance use disorders[5,6,8]; 42% of youth with BPSD experience psychosis.[8] A history of suicide attempts is reported in 22% of children with MDD and 44% of children with BD-I or BD-II.[2]

Family Functioning and Childhood Mood Disorders

Both BPSD and DSD are associated with significant functional impairment including problems with peers, family, and school.[1,2,12] Children with mood disorders experience greater tension between themselves and their parents and experience less maternal warmth than children without mood disorders; these differences may be due in part to parents being more likely to have a mood disorder themselves.[12,13] Family relationships and parenting factors including warmth/hostility, attachment, criticism, and parents' coping are possible contributors to children's mood symptoms.[5,13–16] High levels of criticism in parent-child relationships are associated with lower child social competence, depressive symptoms, and suicidal ideation.[15,16] Several psychotherapeutic interventions have been developed to address these factors.

FAMILY-BASED PSYCHOTHERAPY: A REVIEW OF THE EVIDENCE

As childhood BPSDs and DSDs are not uncommon and are clearly impairing for children and their families, identification of efficacious interventions could significantly benefit public health. Treatment guidelines for BPSD and DSD have been developed and published.[5,17,18] Psychotropic medications are commonly recommended and prescribed. Psychotherapy has also been established as an important component of mood disorder treatment. Psychotherapy provides support to patients and families; helps families to cope with mood disorders and their associated impairments; promotes medication compliance; supports psychological development; improves social, family, and academic functioning; and decreases mood symptoms and rates of relapse.[13,19–22]

With emerging data on the family-related impairments associated with mood disorders, efforts to develop family-based psychotherapies (FBPs) have increased. This article focuses specifically on FBPs for childhood mood disorders that have been examined in RCTs. For purposes of this review, FBP is defined as psychotherapy that regularly involves concurrent participation by a youth and one or more caregivers in therapy sessions. Only studies including children meeting DSM[9,10] mood disorder criteria were included (**Table 1**).

Cognitive Behavioral Therapy

Goodyer and colleagues[23] investigated the efficacy of CBT with parent involvement at the end of each session for adolescents with DSD. CBT components included the following:

- Engagement/goal setting
- Emotional recognition/self-monitoring
- Behavioral activation
- Cognitive restructuring
- Problem-solving and communication skills[23]

Table 1
Randomized controlled trials of family-based therapies for childhood mood disorders

Authors	Participants & Demographics	Diagnoses	Therapists	Measures	Treatment Conditions	Results
Diamond et al,[32] 2010	N = 66, age 12–17 y 17% adolescent boys 74.2% African American	39% MDD, 8% DD; participants selected for elevated depressive symptoms and suicidal ideation	Master's and doctoral level	BD-I, BD-II, SIQ-JR, SSI, DISC	ABFT (12 weekly 60- to 90-min adolescent-parent sessions) (n = 35) EUC (facilitated referrals with ongoing clinical monitoring) (n = 31)	ABFT: faster rate of improvement in suicidal ideation and depressive symptoms with benefits maintained at 3-mo follow-up
Diamond et al,[33] 2002	N = 32, age 13–17 y 22% adolescent boys 31% white, 69% African American	MDD	Master's and doctoral level	BDI, BHS, YSR, SRFF, STAIC, CBCL, HAM-D, K-SADS	ABFT (12 weekly 60- to 90-min adolescent-parent sessions) (n = 16) WLC (n = 16)	ABFT: greater improvement in depressive symptoms per clinician ratings, greater youth-reported improvement in anxiety and family conflict (ds = 0.64–1.3)
Fristad,[46] 2006	N = 20, age 8–11 y 85% boys 90% white	40% BD-I, 35% BD-II, 25% BD-NOS	Doctoral level	EEAC, therapy evaluation form, provider and medication usage grids, MSI	IF-PEP (16 alternating parent and child sessions 50 min each) + TAU (n = 10) WLC + TAU (n = 10)	IF-PEP: greater improvement in family interaction; positive consumer evaluations from parents and children Both groups demonstrated improvements in mood symptoms posttreatment and at 12-mo follow-up

Study	Sample	Diagnoses	Therapist level	Measures	Intervention	Outcomes
Fristad et al,[41] 2002; Fristad et al,[42] 2003; Goldberg-Arnold et al,[43] 1999	N = 35, age 8–11 y, 77% boys, 88.5% white, 2.9% Hispanic, 2.9% African American, 2.9% Southeast Asian, 2.9% American Indian	11% BD-I, 34% BD-II, 17% DD, 37% MDD	Master's and doctoral level	UMDQ, EEAC, SSS, CASA	MF-PEP (6 parent and child group sessions 75 min each) + TAU (n = 18); WLC + TAU (n = 17)	MF-PEP: greater improvement in family interaction and parent knowledge of mood disorders at 2- and 6-mo follow-ups; improved service utilization at 6-mo follow-up; greater improvement in child-reported social support from parents at 6-mo follow-up
Fristad et al,[39] 2009	N = 165, age 8–11 y, 73% boys, 90.9% white, 6.7% African American, 1.8% bi/multiracial, 0.6% Hispanic	38% BD-I, 13% BD-II, 18% BD-NOS, 1% substance-induced mood disorder, 3% MDD, 3% MDD + DD, 3% DD, 1% mood disorder NOS	Master's- and doctoral-level therapists; 12 graduate students as cotherapists	MSI	MF-PEP (8 parent and child group sessions 90 min each) + TAU (n = 78); WLC + TAU (n = 87)	MF-PEP: greater mood symptom improvement at 1-y follow-up (d = 0.53)
Goldstein et al,[27] 2014	N = 20, age 12–18 y, 25% adolescent boys, 80% white, 10% African American, 10% multiracial	15% BD-I, 40% BD-II, 45% BD-NOS	Masters and doctoral level	K-SADS, A-LIFE, PSR, SIQ-Jr, LIFE, CALS	DBT (36 alternating individual child and family skills sessions 60 min each) (n =14); TAU (n = 6)	DBT: significantly fewer severe depressive symptoms over time (d = 0.98); more likely to demonstrate improvement in suicidal ideation; nonsignificant group differences in manic symptoms and emotional dysregulation

(continued on next page)

Table 1
(continued)

Authors	Participants & Demographics	Diagnoses	Therapists	Measures	Treatment Conditions	Results
Goodyer et al,[23] 2007	N = 208, age 11–17 y 26% adolescent boys All living in Manchester or Cambridge, England (no race/ethnicity data reported)	MDD or probable MDD (4 rather than 5 symptoms of MDD with psychosocial impairment)	Doctoral level (psychiatrists and psychologists)	K-SADS, Health of the Nation outcome scale, CDRS-R	CBT (18 individual youth sessions 55 min each over 24 wk + 1 final session at 28 wk, each with parent participation at the end of the session) + SSRI (n = 105) SSRI alone (n = 103)	Both groups demonstrated improvement in depressive symptoms, overall functioning, and suicidality; no apparent group differences.
Luby et al,[29] 2012	N = 43, age 3–7 y 63% boys 86% white, 9% black, 5% other	MDD	Master's and doctoral level	PAPA, PFC-S, HBQ, KIDSEDF, BRIEF, PSI	PCIT-ED (14 parent-child sessions over 12 wk) (n = 25) DEPI (12 parent psychoeducational group sessions of 60 min over 12 wk) (n = 18)	Both groups showed significant declines in depressive severity and in internalizing, depression, and functional impairment domains PCIT-ED: greater improvement in emotion recognition skills (d = 0.83), executive functioning (ds = 0.33–0.50), and parenting stress in the child domain (d = 1.53) and total stress (d = 0.54)

Study	Sample	Diagnosis		Measures	Treatment conditions	Outcomes
Miklowitz et al,[35] 2008	N = 58, age 12–17 y, 43.1% adolescent boys, 89.7% white, 5.2% biracial, 1.7% African American, 1.7% American Indian, 1.7% Asian/Pacific Islander	65.5% BD-I, 10.3% BD-II, 24.1% BD-NOS	Not reported	K-SADS, A-LIFE	FFT-A (21 adolescent-only, parent-only, or family sessions of 50 min) + pharmacotherapy (n = 30) EC (3 family sessions of 50 min each) + pharmacotherapy (n = 28)	FFT-A: more rapid improvement in depressive symptoms, fewer weeks in depressive episodes, more time without depressive symptoms, and greater improvement in depressive symptoms over 2 y. No group differences in rates of recovery from index episode or time to recurrence
Miklowitz et al,[36] 2013	N = 40, age 9–17 y, 57.5% adolescent boys, 90% white, 5% Hispanic ethnicity	42.5% MDD, 7.5% cyclothymic disorder, 50% BD-NOS	Not reported	YMRS, CDRS-R, A-LIFE, PSR, FMSS	FFT-HR (8 weekly + 4 biweekly adolescent-only, parent-only, or family sessions) + as-needed pharmacotherapy (n = 21) FEC (1–2 family sessions) + as-needed pharmacotherapy (n = 19)	FFT-HR: faster improvement of initial mood symptoms, more time in remission, less time with subthreshold mood symptoms, and greater improvement of manic symptoms over 1 y; FFT-HR was more effective in improving mood symptoms for children in more highly critical/conflictual families

(continued on next page)

Table 1
(continued)

Authors	Participants & Demographics	Diagnoses	Therapists	Measures	Treatment Conditions	Results
Sanford et al,[47] 2006	N = 31, age 13–18 y 35.5% adolescent boys All living in Canada (no race/ethnicity data reported)	MDD (12.9% MDD with psychosis)	Not reported	RADS, FAD, ACL, SSAI	FPE (12 sessions of 90 min each at home with all family members who agreed to participate) + TAU (n = 16) TAU (n = 15)	FPE: faster rates of improvement in family functioning, greater improvement in global social function (ds >0.9), depressive symptoms (d = 0.52, 0.64) at the 6- and 9-mo follow-ups
Trowell et al,[30] 2007	N = 72, age 9–15 y 62% boys 87% white, 6% Asian, 6% other	45% MDD, 8% DD, 47% MDD + DD	Not reported	CDI, K-SADS, MFQ, CGAS	SIFT (8–14 family sessions 90 min each) (n = 37) FIPP (16–30 individual child sessions 50 min each + 1 individual parent session for every 2 child sessions) (n = 35)	Both groups showed high response rates and did not differ SIFT: greater decline in child-reported depression at end of treatment but not at 6-mo follow-up

| West et al,[24] 2014 | N = 69, age 7–13 y 58% boys 52% white, 30% African American, 10% Hispanic, 5% American Indian/ Alaskan, 1% American Indian/ Pacific Islander | Bachelor's, master's, + doctoral level | 31.9% BD-I, 5.8% BD-II, 62.3% BD-NOS | K-SADS, CDRS-R, CGI | CFF-CBT (12 weekly 60- to 90-min sessions with the parent, child, or family) + pharmacotherapy (n = 34) TAU + pharmacotherapy (n = 35) | CFF-CBT: reported greater treatment satisfaction, demonstrated greater reductions in parent-reported mania posttreatment (n = 34) and depression posttreatment (d = 0.69) and depression posttreatment (d = 0.55) and at 6-mo follow-up (d = 0.48); nonsignificant differences in global functioning |

Abbreviations: ABFT, Attachment-Based Family Therapy; ACL, Adjective Checklist; A-LIFE, Adolescent Longitudinal Interval Follow-Up Evaluation; BDI, Beck Depression Inventory; BHS, Beck Hopelessness Scale; BRIEF, Behavior Rating Inventory of Executive Function; CALS, Children's Affective Lability Scale; CASA, Child and Adolescent Services Assessment; CBCL, Child Behavior Checklist; CDI, Child Depression Inventory; CDRS-R, Child Depression Rating Scale-Revised; CGAS, Children's Global Assessment Scale; CFF-CBT, child- and family-focused cognitive behavioral therapy; CGI, Children's Global Impressions scale; *d*, Cohen's d, a measure of effect size; DBT, dialectical behavior therapy; DD, dysthymic disorder; DEPI, Developmental Education and Parenting Intervention; DISC, Diagnostic Interview Schedule for Children; EC, educational control; EEAC, Expressed Emotion Adjective Checklist; EUC, enhanced usual care; FAD, Family Assessment Device; FEC, family educational control; FFT-A, family-focused therapy-adolescent; FFT-HR, family-focused therapy-high risk; FIPP, Focused Individual Psychodynamic Psychotherapy; FMSS, Five-Minute Speech Sample; HAM-D, Hamilton Depression Rating Scale; HBQ, Health and Behavior Questionnaire; IF-PEP, Individual-Family Psychoeducational Psychotherapy; KIDSEDF, Penn Emotion Differentiation Test; K-SADS, Kiddie Schedule for Affective Disorders and Schizophrenia; LIFE, Longitudinal Follow-Up Evaluation; MF-PEP, Multi-Family Psychoeducational Psychotherapy; MFQ, Mood and Feelings Questionnaire; MSI, Mood Severity Index; NOS, not otherwise specified; PAPA, Preschool Age Psychiatric Assessment; PCIT-ED, Parent-Child Interaction Therapy-Emotion Development; PFC-S, Preschool Feelings Checklist-Scale Version; PSI, Parenting Stress Index; PSR, Psychiatric Status Screening; RADS, Reynolds Adolescent Depression Scale; SIFT, Systems Integrative Family Therapy; SIQ-Jr, Suicidal Ideation Questionnaire-Junior; SRF, Self-Report of Family Functioning; SSAI, Structured Social Adjustment Interview; SSI, Scale for Suicidal Ideation; SSRI, selective serotonin reuptake inhibitor; SSS, Social Support Scale; STAIC, State-Trait Anxiety Inventory for Children; TAU, treatment as usual; UMDQ, Understanding Mood Disorders Questionnaire; WLC, wait list control; YMRS, Young Mania Rating Scale; YSR, Youth Self-Report.

In a study of 208 adolescents who received a 28-week intervention of either 19 sessions of CBT of 55 minutes each plus a selective serotonin reuptake inhibitor (SSRI) or an SSRI alone, both groups showed significant improvements in depressive symptoms, overall functioning, and suicidality. CBT did not seem to provide benefit beyond that provided by SSRI alone.

Child- and family-focused CBT (CFF-CBT) was designed to address symptoms and impairment related to childhood BPSD. CFF-CBT includes 12 weekly 60- to 90-minute child, parent, or family sessions and 7 treatment components that spell "RAINBOW":

1. Routine: developing consistent daily routines
2. Affect regulation: mood identification, coping strategies
3. I can do it!: improving self-esteem
4. No negative thoughts/live in the now: cognitive restructuring and mindfulness
5. Be a good friend/balanced lifestyle: learning social skills and parent self-care
6. Oh how do we solve this problem?: learning problem-solving/communication skills
7. Ways to find support: enhancing social support[24]

In a study of 69 children with BPSD who received either CFF-CBT or treatment as usual (TAU), the CFF-CBT group attended more therapy sessions and reported greater satisfaction with treatment. CFF-CBT yielded greater reduction in parent-reported mania posttreatment and depressive symptoms posttreatment and at 6-month follow-up.[24] This result suggests that involving families in CBT-based therapy for BPSD may be efficacious in mood symptom reduction.

Dialectical Behavior Therapy

Dialectical behavior therapy (DBT), originally developed to treat adults with borderline personality disorder, has been modified to treat BPSD and suicidality in adolescents.[25] In the first 6 months of DBT for adolescent BPSD, adolescents attend 24 weekly 60-minute sessions alternating between family and individual sessions. In the last 6 months, adolescents attend 1 family session and 1 individual session monthly to review skills and consolidate gains.

- Family skills training: psychoeducation about DBT and BPSD; mindfulness, distress tolerance, emotion regulation, and social skills
- Adolescent individual therapy sessions: problem-solving strategies
- Skills coaching: therapist available by phone for skills coaching as needed[26]

Goldstein and colleagues[27] examined the efficacy of DBT for 20 adolescents with BPSD compared with TAU in ameliorating mood symptoms. Although both treatment groups demonstrated high acceptability, adolescents in DBT attended more sessions and demonstrated greater improvement in depressive (but not manic) symptoms and suicidal ideation.[27] Thus, DBT seems to be a promising treatment of adolescent BPSD, particularly for depressive symptoms.

Parent-Child Interaction Therapy

Parent-Child Interaction Therapy (PCIT), a therapy that uses modeling and in-session coaching to promote positive parent-child relationships and firm yet warm parenting, is an effective treatment for young children with disruptive behavior disorders.[28] Luby and colleagues[29] added a module addressing emotion recognition and regulation to the core PCIT to treat preschoolers with MDD (PCIT-Emotion Development

[PCIT-ED]). PCIT-ED is delivered in 14 sessions over 12 weeks and includes the following modules:

- Child-directed interaction: positive-play techniques to improve the parent-child relationship
- Parent-directed interaction: effective commands and firm, nonpunitive behavior management strategies
- Emotion development (novel): emotion competence and regulation strategies; coaching parent to help the child identify and regulate emotions

Luby and colleagues[29] examined the efficacy of PCIT-ED compared with Developmental Education and Parenting Intervention (12 weekly 60-minute parent group sessions focused on child social and emotional development) in 43 preschoolers with MDD. Both groups demonstrated improved depressive symptom severity; PCIT-ED, however, was more efficacious in improving executive functioning and emotion recognition skills. PCIT-ED was the only identified FBP for preschoolers with mood disorders.

Family Systems Therapy

Trowell and colleagues[30] tested the hypothesis that Focused Individual Psychodynamic Psychotherapy (FIPP) is more efficacious than Systems Integrative Family Therapy (SIFT) in treating childhood depression using a 9-month RCT including 72 youth aged 9 to 15 years.[30] FIPP focuses on relationships, life stresses, and dysfunctional attachments, whereas SIFT focuses on family dysfunction without explicit attention to unresolved intrapsychic conflicts. In the study,[30] FIPP included 16 to 30 individual child sessions of 50 minutes each with 1 parent session for every 2 child sessions. SIFT involved 8 to 14 family sessions of 90 minutes each. Youth in both groups demonstrated high response rates. Those in SIFT reported greater reduction of depressive symptoms posttreatment, although SIFT and FIPP were no longer significantly different at the 6-month follow-up assessment.[30] Thus, it is unclear whether systems-based family therapy might be more efficacious than individual psychodynamic therapy.

Attachment-Based Family Therapy (ABFT) is derived from theory suggesting that family relationships can precipitate, exacerbate, or serve as a protective factor for depression and suicide.[31] ABFT is a process-oriented, emotion-focused treatment[32] including 12 weekly 60- to 90-minute adolescent-parent sessions consisting of 5 tasks or phases:

1. Relational reframe: strengthening relationships
2. Adolescent alliance: 1 to 2 adolescent-only sessions identifying family conflicts that may have contributed to depressed mood
3. Parent alliance: 1 to 2 parent-only sessions teaching emotion-focused parenting skills to improve parents' empathy and insight
4. Reattachment: together, parent or parents and adolescent discuss identified problems and learn new communication, problem-solving, and coping skills
5. Competency: improving the adolescent's autonomy while maintaining a healthy relationship with parents.[32,33]

In an RCT, 32 adolescents with MDD were randomized into ABFT or wait list control (WLC). Those in ABFT demonstrated greater improvement in clinician-rated depressive symptoms and youth-reported anxiety and family conflict.[33] Another RCT examined the efficacy of ABFT compared with enhanced usual care (facilitated referrals with ongoing clinical monitoring) in treating 66 youth with depressive symptoms and suicidal ideation (47% had DSD). Youth in ABFT demonstrated faster rates of improvement in suicidal ideation and depressive symptoms with benefits maintained at 3-month follow-up assessment.[32] Taken together, these results suggest that structured, goal-oriented family therapy may be efficacious in treating adolescent depression and suicidality.

Family Psychoeducation Plus Skill Building

Family-Focused Treatment for Adolescents (FFT-A) includes 21 (12 weekly, 6 biweekly, and 3 monthly) 50-minute adolescent, parent, or family sessions over 9 months.[34,35] FFT-A was developed to treat adolescent BPSD and includes involvement from the youth, parents, and siblings. The components are as follows:

- FPE about the nature and course of BPSD and evidence-based treatments
- Communication skill building
- Problem-solving skills training

A total of 58 families of adolescents with BPSD were randomized to FFT-A and pharmacotherapy or to enhanced care (3 weekly 50-minute family sessions) and pharmacotherapy. Youth whose families received FFT-A demonstrated faster improvement in depressive symptoms, spent less time in depressive episodes, and demonstrated greater reduction in depressive symptom severity over 2 years.[35] Miklowitz and colleagues[36,37] modified FFT to treat younger children at high risk for BD (children with diagnoses of MDD, BD-NOS, or cyclothymia with parents diagnosed with BD-I or BD-II; Family-Focused Therapy-High Risk [FFT-HR]). FFT-HR includes 12 (8 weekly, 4 biweekly) adolescent, parent, or family sessions conducted over 4 months. A total of 40 children were randomized to FFT-HR or a family education control (1–2 family sessions). Those in the FFT-HR arm recovered more quickly from their initial mood symptoms, spent more time in remission, and demonstrated greater reduction in manic symptoms over 1 year.[36]

Multi-Family Psychoeducational Psychotherapy (MF-PEP) is a group intervention including 8 concurrent parent and child sessions of 90 minutes each developed as an adjunctive treatment for children with DSD or BPSD.[38] This intervention incorporates psychoeducation, family systems concepts, and CBT techniques. Sessions begin with parents and children together to review between-session projects and end with children reviewing their session content with parents. Key components are the following:

- Parent and child psychoeducation about symptoms and evidence-based treatments
- Facilitated social support
- Emotion regulation skills training
- Strategies for navigating the mental health system
- Altering maladaptive family interaction patterns
- Cognitive restructuring
- Family problem-solving and communication skill building.[38]

MF-PEP plus TAU was compared with WLC plus TAU in 165 children with DSD or BPSD aged 8 to 11 years. The MF-PEP group demonstrated greater improvement in mood severity,[39,40] and participation in MF-PEP improved the quality of services that children received, mediated by parents' treatment beliefs.[41] In a pilot RCT, MF-PEP demonstrated greater improvements in family interactions and knowledge of mood disorders compared with WLC.[41–43] In addition, comorbid behavior and anxiety disorders did not impede improvement in mood,[44,45] and behavioral symptoms improved with treatment.[44] These findings suggests that MF-PEP is efficacious in treating mood disorders and improving service engagement. An individual-family version of MF-PEP, called Individual-Family Psychoeducational Psychotherapy (IF-PEP),[38] has demonstrated a medium effect size in ameliorating mood symptom severity for children with BPSD.[46] The efficacy of IF-PEP among children with DSD is currently being evaluated in an RCT.

Sanford and colleagues[47] conducted a small pilot study of FPE involving 12 family sessions of 90 minutes each and 1 booster session conducted in the homes of 31 adolescents with MDD (aged 13–18 years). The following are the goals of FPE:

- Increasing family knowledge about depression and its impact on families
- Improving family communication
- Enhancing coping and problem-solving skills[47]

Adolescents were randomized to FPE plus TAU or TAU alone. FPE demonstrated faster rates of improvement in family functioning and greater improvement in social functioning and depressive symptoms.[47] FPE seems to be a promising treatment for youth with MDD; replication in a larger RCT would provide more support of its efficacy.

FFT, MF-PEP, and FPE each demonstrate efficacy in treating mood symptoms of youth with DSD or BPSD with FPE plus skill building.

TREATMENT COMPLICATIONS AND SUGGESTED ADAPTATIONS

Complex presentation and comorbidity is common among children with mood disorders. Suggestions for how to manage treatment complications are presented in **Table 2**.

The following case illustrates use of IF-PEP in the treatment of an 8-year-old girl, Anna (identifying information has been altered to protect confidentiality), in the context of a larger treatment study.

Table 2	
Strategies for managing treatment complications	
Complication	**Suggested Strategies**
Treatment resistance	• Per treatment guidelines, refer for a medication evaluation or consult with prescribing physician • Consult with school personnel to address symptom management at school • Assess adherence to psychotherapy and medication
Comorbidity	• Because evidence-based treatments for some common comorbid disorders use similar strategies as those discussed in this review, evidence-based treatments for mood disorders may ameliorate some comorbid symptoms as well • Supplement with evidence-based strategies to treat comorbid conditions as necessary (eg, medication management for ADHD, exposure-response prevention for anxiety disorders) • Consult with the prescribing physician or school personnel, as needed • If another disorder is primary, consider addressing those symptoms first • For substance and autism spectrum disorders, simultaneously begin treatment of those conditions • Develop safety/crisis plans early in treatment to manage suicidality
Relapse	• Conclude therapy with a thorough review of newly learned skills • Use booster sessions to review skills and prevent relapse • Provide psychoeducation to parents and youth about relapse early in treatment; coach them to notice warning signs and recognize when further treatment is needed

CLINICAL CASE EXAMPLE
Presentation

At intake, Anna presented with dysphoric and irritable mood, anhedonia, decreased concentration, and feelings of worthlessness (eg, saying that she was stupid or that she hated herself) and significant psychotic symptoms, including hallucinations, delusions, and disorganized speech. Anna commented that she could see people's organs and bad spirits. Anna's mother, Ms Jones, described Anna as sad and tearful all day, every day, and noted that Anna occasionally experienced passive suicidal ideation. Per Ms Jones, Anna had difficulty maintaining friendships and was often physically aggressive toward her younger brother. Anna often worried about her future as well as the health of her family members and finances. Anna's intelligence quotient was in the average range. The family was advised that pharmacotherapy is the first-line treatment of psychosis, but Ms Jones was adamantly opposed, preferring FBP instead.

Diagnoses

Thorough assessment of Anna's presenting concerns, history, and family functioning through parent and child interviews revealed symptoms consistent with schizoaffective disorder, depressive type, and generalized anxiety disorder. Parent- and child-reported inattention and hyperactivity were better accounted for by Anna's psychotic symptoms than by an independent ADHD diagnosis; treatment included a plan to monitor these symptoms to further clarify whether a separate ADHD diagnosis was warranted.

Developmental History

Anna was delivered vaginally at full term without complications and was reportedly healthy at birth. As an infant, Anna was diagnosed with reactive airway disease, and she had continued to use an inhaler as needed. Anna reportedly met all developmental milestones within healthy limits.

Treatment Summary

Anna and Ms Jones attended 10 child sessions and 10 parent sessions over 3 months. Rapport was easily established with Ms Jones. Although guarded initially, Anna quickly warmed up in therapy. With their therapist, Anna and Ms Jones developed 3 treatment goals: (1) reduction in the frequency and intensity of Anna's depressed and irritable moods and psychotic symptoms, (2) improvement in Anna's self-esteem, and (3) improvement in Anna's social relationships. The therapist met with Anna and Ms Jones together at the beginning of each child session to assess Anna's functioning and address any new concerns. The 3 also met at the end of each session for Anna to share with Ms Jones the content of that day's session and to aid Ms Jones in facilitating Anna's skills generalization.

Treatment began by providing psychoeducation regarding depression and psychosis to Anna and teaching her to identify and rate the intensity of her feelings in order to improve her ability to recognize and communicate her mood states. Anna practiced identifying her feelings at the beginning of each subsequent session. Next, to improve Anna's self-esteem, Anna learned to differentiate herself from her symptoms. In future sessions, Anna was encouraged to identify triggers of different feelings and to develop a "tool kit" of pleasant and fun activities she could use as coping strategies. She was asked to practice using these strategies and to note their effectiveness in improving her mood between sessions. There was additional focus on triggers of psychosis and effective coping strategies. The therapist assisted Anna in identifying ways to communicate with Ms Jones and school staff about her mood and psychotic symptoms to elicit their support in coping. Anna was then taught to recognize the relationship among thoughts, feelings, and behaviors and was presented with age-appropriate examples of cognitive restructuring. With assistance from Ms Jones, Anna practiced identifying negative automatic thoughts, evaluating their accuracy, and developing more balanced thinking at home. Anna then learned problem-solving skills including concrete steps to solve interpersonal problems. Last, Anna was taught strategies to improve nonverbal and verbal communication.

Ms Jones' sessions began with psychoeducation about mood disorders, psychotic disorders, and their evidenced-based treatments. Throughout the course of therapy, there was a specific focus on pharmacotherapy for psychosis and frequent discussion of Anna's likely need for additional treatment. Ms Jones was encouraged to monitor, rate, and record Anna's moods and behaviors between sessions. The therapist discussed possible school-based interventions for Anna and provided guidance to Ms Jones in communicating Anna's mental health needs to Anna's school. Parent sessions then focused on parenting strategies to help manage Anna's mood and coping strategies for Ms Jones to use. The relationship between thoughts, feelings, and actions was discussed, and Ms Jones was encouraged to use cognitive reframing strategies. The therapist then reviewed family problem-solving and communication skills with Ms Jones.

The final parent and child session involved a review of skills learned in therapy, including strategies to prevent relapse. At the end of treatment, both Anna and Ms Jones reported feeling that they better understood Anna's symptoms and how to manage them. Ms Jones reported greater willingness to consider psychotropic medication and scheduled a medication consultation.

Over the course of treatment, Anna became better able to identify her feelings and recognize her psychotic symptoms. As part of treatment, the therapist provided Anna's school staff with information about her symptoms and diagnoses and, per Ms Jones and Anna, the staff responded to Anna's symptoms in a more supportive manner. Consequently, Anna was able to recognize psychotic symptoms earlier, notify a teacher, and use coping strategies to manage her mood. Ms Jones reported that Anna was also able to use these skills at home, resulting in fewer conflicts with her mother and siblings. Although Anna continued to experience psychotic symptoms, her depressive symptoms improved over the course of treatment. An independent evaluator rated Anna's depression as moderate at the beginning of treatment, decreasing to borderline at the end of treatment. To address remaining symptoms after completing IF-PEP sessions that were included in the treatment study, Anna was referred for medication management and ongoing therapy.

SUMMARY

Given the impairment and risks associated with childhood mood disorders, effective treatment is essential for child, family, and public health. Family-based interventions address family-related correlates of mood disorders and the impact mood symptoms can have on family functioning. Evidence is mounting for their benefit in treating children with DSD and BPSD. Research examining treatment moderators, benefit of family-focused treatment compared with individual approaches, family-focused treatment for younger children, and the effects of mood disorder treatments on comorbid diagnoses will further allow for effective, evidence-based yet individualized treatment for children with mood disorders.

REFERENCES

1. Birmaher B, Arbelaez C, Brent D. Course and outcome of child and adolescent major depressive disorder. Child Adolesc Psychiatr Clin N Am 2002;11:619–37.
2. Youngstrom EA, Birmaher B, Findling RL. Pediatric bipolar disorder: validity, phenomenology and recommendations for diagnosis. Bipolar Disord 2008;10: 194–214.
3. Van Meter AR, Moreira AL, Youngstrom EA. Meta-analysis of epidemiologic studies of pediatric bipolar disorder. J Clin Psychiatry 2011;72:1250–6.
4. Costello EJ, Erkanli A, Angold A. Is there an epidemic of child or adolescent depression? J Child Psychol Psychiatry 2006;47:1263–71.
5. Birmaher B, Brent D, AACAP Work Group on Quality Issues. Practice parameter for the assessment and treatment of children and adolescents with depressive disorders. J Am Acad Child Adolesc Psychiatry 2007;46:1503–26.
6. Kovacs M. Presentation and course of major depressive disorder during childhood and later years of the life span. J Am Acad Child Adolesc Psychiatry 1996;35:705–15.
7. Geller B, Tillman R, Craney JL, et al. Four-year prospective outcome and natural history of mania in children with prepubertal and early adolescent bipolar disorder phenotype. Arch Gen Psychiatry 2004;61:459–67.
8. Kowatch RA, Youngstrom EA, Danielyan A, et al. Review and meta-analysis of the phenomenology and clinical characteristics of mania in children and adolescents. Bipolar Disord 2005;7:483–96.
9. American Psychiatric Association. Diagnostic and statistical manual of mental disorders: DSM-IV-TR. Washington, DC: American Psychiatric Association; 2000.
10. American Psychiatric Association. Diagnostic and statistical manual of mental disorders: DSM-5. Washington, DC: American Psychiatric Association; 2013.
11. Axelson DA, Birmaher B, Strober MA, et al. Course of subthreshold bipolar disorder in youth: diagnostic progression from bipolar disorder not otherwise specified. J Am Acad Child Adolesc Psychiatry 2011;50:1001–16.e3.
12. Fristad MA, Frazier TW, Youngstrom EA, et al. What differentiates children visiting outpatient mental health services with bipolar spectrum disorder from children with other psychiatric diagnoses? Bipolar Disord 2012;14:497–506.
13. Stark KD, Banneyer KN, Wang LA, et al. Child and adolescent depression in the family. Couple Family Psychol 2012;1:161–84.
14. Coville AL, Miklowitz DJ, Taylor DO, et al. Correlates of high expressed emotion attitudes among parents of bipolar adolescents. J Clin Psychol 2008;64: 438–49.
15. Ellis AJ, Portnoff LC, Axelson DA, et al. Parental expressed emotion and suicidal ideation in adolescents with bipolar disorder. Psychiatry Res 2014;216:213–6.
16. Tompson MC, Pierre CB, Boger KD, et al. Maternal depression, maternal expressed emotion, and youth psychopathology. J Abnorm Child Psychol 2010; 38:105–17.
17. Kowatch RA, Fristad M, Birmaher B, et al. Treatment guidelines for children and adolescents with bipolar disorder. J Am Acad Child Adolesc Psychiatry 2005;44: 213–35.
18. McClellan J, Kowatch R, Findling RL, Work Group on Quality Issues. Practice parameter for the assessment and treatment of children and adolescents with bipolar disorder. J Am Acad Child Adolesc Psychiatry 2007;46:107–25.
19. Jones S. Psychotherapy of bipolar disorder: a review. J Affect Disord 2004;80: 101–14.

20. David-Ferdon C, Kaslow NJ. Evidence-based psychosocial treatments for child and adolescent depression. J Clin Child Adolesc Psychol 2008;37:62–104.
21. Fristad MA, MacPherson HA. Evidence-based psychosocial treatments for child and adolescent bipolar spectrum disorders. J Clin Child Adolesc Psychol 2014; 43:339–55.
22. Lauder SD, Berk M, Castle DJ, et al. The role of psychotherapy in bipolar disorder. Med J Aust 2010;193:31–5.
23. Goodyer I, Dubicka B, Wilkinson P, et al. Selective serotonin reuptake inhibitors (SSRIs) and routine specialist care with and without cognitive behaviour therapy in adolescents with major depression: randomised controlled trial. BMJ 2007;335:142.
24. West AE, Weinstein SM, Peters AT, et al. Child-and family-focused cognitive-behavioral therapy for pediatric bipolar disorder: a randomized clinical trial. J Am Acad Child Adolesc Psychiatry 2014;53:1168–78.
25. Miller AL, Rathus JH, Linehan M. Dialectical behavior therapy with suicidal adolescents. New York: Guilford Press; 2007.
26. Goldstein TR, Axelson DA, Birmaher B, et al. Dialectical behavior therapy for adolescents with bipolar disorder: a 1-year open trial. J Am Acad Child Adolesc Psychiatry 2007;46:820–30.
27. Goldstein TR, Fersch-Podrat RK, Rivera M, et al. Dialectical behavior therapy for adolescents with bipolar disorder: results from a pilot randomized trial. J Child Adolesc Psychopharmacol 2015;25(2):140–9.
28. Thomas R, Zimmer-Gembeck MJ. Behavioral outcomes of parent-child interaction therapy and triple P—positive parenting program: a review and meta-analysis. J Abnorm Child Psychol 2007;35:475–95.
29. Luby J, Lenze S, Tillman R. A novel early intervention for preschool depression: findings from a pilot randomized controlled trial. J Child Psychol Psychiatry 2012;53:313–22.
30. Trowell J, Joffe I, Campbell J, et al. Childhood depression: a place for psychotherapy: an outcome study comparing individual psychodynamic psychotherapy and family therapy. Eur Child Adolesc Psychiatry 2007;16:157–67.
31. Joiner TE, Coyne JC. The interactional nature of depression: advances in interpersonal approaches. Washington, DC: American Psychological Association; 1999.
32. Diamond GS, Wintersteen MB, Brown GK, et al. Attachment-based family therapy for adolescents with suicidal ideation: a randomized controlled trial. J Am Acad Child Adolesc Psychiatry 2010;49:122–31.
33. Diamond GS, Reis BF, Diamond GM, et al. Attachment-based family therapy for depressed adolescents: a treatment development study. J Am Acad Child Adolesc Psychiatry 2002;41:1190–6.
34. Miklowitz DJ, George EL, Axelson DA, et al. Family-focused treatment for adolescents with bipolar disorder. J Affect Disord 2004;82:S113–28.
35. Miklowitz DJ, Axelson DA, Birmaher B, et al. Family-focused treatment for adolescents with bipolar disorder: results of a 2-year randomized trial. J Affect Disord 2008;82:1053–61.
36. Miklowitz DJ, Schneck CD, Singh MK, et al. Early intervention for symptomatic youth at risk for bipolar disorder: a randomized trial of family-focused therapy. J Am Acad Child Adolesc Psychiatry 2013;52:121–31.
37. Miklowitz DJ, Chang KD, Taylor DO, et al. Early psychosocial intervention for youth at risk for bipolar I or II disorder: a one-year treatment development trial: youth at risk for bipolar disorder. Bipolar Disord 2011;13:67–75.
38. Fristad MA, Goldberg-Arnold JS, Leffler JM. Psychotherapy for children with bipolar and depressive disorders. New York: Guilford Press; 2011.

39. Fristad MA, Verducci JS, Walters K, et al. Impact of multifamily psychoeducational psychotherapy in treating children aged 8 to 12 years with mood disorders. Arch Gen Psychiatry 2009;66:1013–20.

40. Mendenhall AN, Fristad MA, Early TJ. Factors influencing service utilization and mood symptom severity in children with mood disorders: effects of multifamily psychoeducation groups (MFPGs). J Consult Clin Psychol 2009;77:463–73.

41. Fristad MA, Goldberg-Arnold JS, Gavazzi SM. Multifamily psychoeducation groups (MFPG) for families of children with bipolar disorder. Bipolar Disord 2002;4:254–62.

42. Fristad MA, Goldberg-Arnold JS, Gavazzi SM. Multi-family psychoeducation groups in the treatment of children with mood disorders. J Marital Fam Ther 2003;29:491–504.

43. Goldberg-Arnold JS, Fristad MA, Gavazzi SM. Family psychoeducation: giving caregivers what they want and need. Fam Relat 1999;48:411.

44. Boylan K, MacPherson HA, Fristad MA. Examination of disruptive behavior outcomes and moderation in a randomized psychotherapy trial for mood disorders. J Am Acad Child Adolesc Psychiatry 2013;52:699–708.

45. Cummings CM, Fristad MA. Anxiety in children with mood disorders: a treatment help or hindrance? J Abnorm Child Psychol 2012;40:339–51.

46. Fristad MA. Psychoeducational treatment for school-aged children with bipolar disorder. Dev Psychopathol 2006;18:1289–306.

47. Sanford M, Boyle M, McCleary L, et al. A pilot study of adjunctive family psychoeducation in adolescent major depression: feasibility and treatment effect. J Am Acad Child Adolesc Psychiatry 2006;45:386–95.

Family-Based Treatment of Pediatric Obsessive-Compulsive Disorder
Clinical Considerations and Application

Lindsay M. Anderson, MA[a], Jennifer B. Freeman, PhD[b],
Martin E. Franklin, PhD[c], Jeffrey J. Sapyta, PhD[d],*

KEYWORDS

- Family-based treatment • Obsessive-compulsive disorder • Family accommodation
- Cognitive-behavioral family-based treatment • Pediatric OCD

KEY POINTS

- Pediatric obsessive-compulsive disorder (OCD) can be effectively treated with a family-based approach.
- Family-based cognitive-behavioral therapy works by providing coping strategies, parent training practices for relevant caregivers, routine implementation of exposure and response prevention, and systematic reduction of OCD family accommodation.
- Therapists first model then coach parents in more adaptive responses to OCD symptoms, which often builds skills on how to manage their own anxiety and behavioral responses to OCD.
- Contextual family processes, including family accommodation, family dysfunction, family problem solving, and communication styles, are identified and addressed throughout treatment.
- Therapeutic goals include increased flexibility for individual and family behavioral responses to OCD symptoms.
- Humor and creativity can be extremely beneficial.

The authors have nothing to disclose.
[a] Department of Psychology & Neuroscience, Duke University, 2608 Erwin Road, Suite 300, Durham, NC 27705, USA; [b] Department of Psychiatry and Human Behavior, Warren Alpert Medical School of Brown University, Providence, RI 02912, USA; [c] Department of Psychiatry, University of Pennsylvania Medical School, 3535 Market Street, 6th Floor Philadelphia, PA 19104, USA; [d] Department of Psychiatry and Behavioral Sciences, Duke University School of Medicine, 2608 Erwin Road, Suite 300, Durham, NC 27705, USA
* Corresponding author.
E-mail address: jeffrey.sapyta@duke.edu

Child Adolesc Psychiatric Clin N Am 24 (2015) 535–555
http://dx.doi.org/10.1016/j.chc.2015.02.003
1056-4993/15/$ – see front matter © 2015 Elsevier Inc. All rights reserved.

childpsych.theclinics.com

Abbreviations	
ADIS	Anxiety Disorders Interview Schedule
CBT	Cognitive-behavioral therapy
CY-BOCS	Children's Yale-Brown Obsessive Compulsive Scale
ERP	Exposure and response prevention
FB-CBT	Family-based cognitive-behavioral therapy
FIT	Family inclusive treatment
OCD	Obsessive-compulsive disorder
PFIT	Positive family interaction therapy
SRI	Serotonin reuptake inhibitor

OVERVIEW: NATURE OF THE PROBLEM

Obsessive-compulsive disorder (OCD) is a serious pediatric psychological condition, with childhood prevalence estimates between 1% and 3%.[1–4] The time-consuming and distressing nature of obsessions and compulsions observed in the context of OCD often results in significant disruption in school, social, and family functioning.[5,6] The familial context is an especially important consideration of OCD in children because family factors affect both the development and maintenance of OCD, often with deleterious effects on family relationships and interactions.[7] Family members play an integral part in the treatment of pediatric OCD, including helping children follow through with treatment tasks, extricating themselves from OCD rituals, and broadening family-based behavioral responses to OCD.[7] Indeed, both research and clinical experience indicate that to effectively treat OCD in children and adolescents, families must be involved.

A review of the current literature (**Table 1**, see later discussion) indicates that treatments with family-based components demonstrate large effect sizes. In fact, the more family-based intervention used the more improvement in symptoms and functioning.[22] This is unsurprising given that nearly all families engage in accommodation of OCD.[23–25] Accommodation is a family-based phenomenon that warrants family-based intervention to curb the negative impact on symptoms and reduce distress.

This article aims to describe the clinical application of family-based treatment of pediatric OCD. Three broad areas are discussed: (1) family factors associated with OCD in youth, (2) the current family-based treatment literature for pediatric OCD, and (3) clinical application of family-based treatment in pediatric OCD.

Family and Contextual Factors Observed in Pediatric Obsessive-Compulsive Disorder

Several contextual and family process factors have been found to contribute to the development and maintenance of anxiety and OCD symptoms.

Family accommodation

Family accommodation is characterized by actions taken by family members to either avoid OCD-related triggers or facilitate completion of compulsions. Accommodation can be achieved by actively participating in rituals, offering reassurance, or attempting to decrease the child's anxiety by yielding other family priorities to OCD demands.[25,26] Family engagement in OCD accommodation is strikingly ubiquitous, with some studies reporting more than 97% of reporters acknowledging accommodation, most occurring on a daily basis.[23–25] Despite being well-intentioned and seemingly pragmatic, family accommodation can exacerbate symptoms of OCD by reinforcing compulsive behaviors.

Table 1
Empirical studies evaluating family-based treatment of pediatric obsessive-compulsive disorder

Study	Number of Subjects	Mean Age (Range)	Design	Family-Based Intervention Elements	% Parent Involvement	Primary Outcome Measures	Results	Effect Size
Waters et al,[8] 2001	7	Not reported (10–13 y)	Open: child CBT + parent skills training + family review	PE, reduction of OCD involvement, family support of ERP, increase problem solving	50	• ADIS • CY-BOCS • NIMH GOCS • FAS • M-FAD	• 86% no longer met criteria • 60% reduction in CY-BOCS • 60% reduction in NIMH GOCS • Reduction in family accommodation • No change in family functioning	Sample too small
Grunes et al,[9] 2001	28	28.5 y (8–67 y)	Randomized: ERP vs ERP + FI	Family member in 8-wk FI group (90 min): PE, cotherapist, support, coping skills	~67	• CY-BOCS	• FI-group: 31% reduction in obsessions, 25% reduction in compulsions • ERP-only group: 7% reduction obsessions, 11% reduction compulsions	FI-group: 1.1[+] (Y-BOCS)
Freeman et al,[10] 2003	4	6.75 y (4–11 y)	Open pilot: FB-CBT	PE, parent training, family treatment, ERP	100	• CY-BOCS	• 88% reduction in symptoms ◦ Pretreatment mean = 26 (SD = 4) ◦ Posttreatment mean = 3 (SD = 2)	Sample too small

(continued on next page)

Table 1
(continued)

Study	Number of Subjects	Mean Age (Range)	Design	Family-Based Intervention Elements	% Parent Involvement	Primary Outcome Measures	Results	Effect Size
Barrett et al,[11] 2005 (12-mo, 18-mo follow-up Barrett et al,[12] 2004)	48	13.85 y (7–17 y)	Individual vs group CBFT	See Barrett et al,[12] 2004	~45	• ADIS (diagnosis-free) • CY-BOCS + NIMH GOCS • Predictors of long-term outcomes	• 70% individual CBFT, 70% group CBFT, 84% (no significant difference) • Gains maintained 12 mo, 18 mo, no significant differences between groups • Higher pretreatment severity and higher family dysfunction predicted worse long-term outcomes	2.84[+] (CY-BOCS) 2.76[+] (CY-BOCS)
Martin & Thienemann,[13] 2005	11	11.3 y (8–14 y)	Open: group CBT – Child, parent groups met concurrently then convened	Parent-group mirrored child group (adapted from March & Mulle,[14] 1998)	60	• CY-BOCS • CGI-I • GOCS • COIS-R	• 25% improvement • Ratings "much improved" • Ratings from clinical to subclinical • 44% total functional improvement	0.98

| Storch et al,[15] 2007 | 40 | 13.3 y (7–17 y) | Randomized comparison: Weekly vs intensive FB-CBT | At least 1 parent attended all sessions | 100 | • CY-BOCS
• CGI-S
• CGI-I
• Remission status (no diagnosis via ADIS and CY-BOCS≤10) | • Significant improvement, no difference between groups
• Intensive less impaired immediate posttreatment, effect did not hold at follow-up
• No significant difference in response rate 90% intensive, 65% weekly
• No significant differences at posttherapy or follow-up
  ○ Posttherapy 75% intensive, 50% weekly
  ○ Follow-up 72% intensive, 77% weekly | Intensive: 2.72 (CY-BOCS)
Weekly: 1.73 (CY-BOCS) |

(continued on next page)

Table 1
(continued)

Study	Number of Subjects	Mean Age (Range)	Design	Family-Based Intervention Elements	% Parent Involvement	Primary Outcome Measures	Results	Effect Size
Freeman et al,[16] 2008	42	7.11 y (4–8 y)	Randomized comparison: FB-CBT or FB-RT	PE, parent training, ERP, family treatment	100	• CY-BOCS (total score) • CY-BOCS (remission≤12) • CGI-I (remission: very much or much improved)	• ITT: no significant difference but CBT moderate effect size (d = 0.53) • Completer: CBT 69%, RT 20% • ITT: CBT 50%, RT 20% • Completer: CBT 69%, RT 40% (n.s.) • ITT: CBT: 50%, RT 40% (n.s.)	0.53 (FB-CBT over FB-RT)
O'Leary et al,[17] 2009 (7-y follow-up Barrett et al,[12] 2004)	38	18.4 y (13–24 y)	Individual vs group CBFT	See Barrett et al,[12] 2004	~45	• ADIS (diagnosis-free) • CY-BOCS + NIMH GOCS	• Individual CBFT 79%, group CBFT 95% (no significant difference) • Gains maintained at 7-y (most without interim treatment)	3.26+ (CY-BOCS)
Storch et al,[48] 2010	30	13.4 y (7–19 y)	Open: Intensive FB-CBT (medication nonresponders)	POTS CBT adapted for parent attendance	100	• CY-BOCS • CY-BOCS (clinical improvement: 30% reduction) • Remission: ADIS-IV≤3, CY-BOCS<10	• 54% reduction in symptoms • 80% participants clinically improved • 57% participants remission posttreatment	2.37 (CY-BOCS) 2.91 (CGI-S) 0.75 (COIS-P) 0.72 (COIS-C)

Study	N	Age	Design	Intervention	Sessions	Measures	Outcomes	Effect Size
Peris & Piacentini,[42] 2013	20	12.5 y (8–17 y)	Pilot Randomized: Individual CBT vs individual CBT + PFIT (12 individual CBT + 6 family sessions)	PFIT: addressed familial blame or conflict, enhanced family cohesion, emotion regulation, problem-solving	ST ~30 PFIT ~33	• CGI-I (responder:<3) • CY-BOCS (remission≤10)	• ST 40%, PFIT 70% (d = 0.65) ∘ Maintained 3-mo follow-up • ST 20%, PFIT 50% • PFIT: decreased accommodation, blame, family conflict	0.65 (CYBOCS) favoring PFIT
Barrett et al,[12] 2004	77	10.75 y (individual CBFT) 12.9 y (group CBFT) 11.75 y (waitlist) (7–17 y)	RCT: individual CBFT, group CBFT, or waitlist	PE, problem-solving skills, strategies to reduce involvement in child's symptoms, family support of ERP	~45	• ADIS (diagnosis-free) • CY-BOCS • NIMH GOCS	• 88% individual CBFT, 76% group CBFT, 22% waitlist • 65% reduction individual CBFT, 61% group CBFT, both significantly better than waitlist (0% reduction) • 60% decrease individual CBFT, 63% group CBFT, both significantly better than waitlist (0% decrease)	2.76 (CY-BOCS)

(continued on next page)

Table 1
(continued)

Study	Number of Subjects	Mean Age (Range)	Design	Family-Based Intervention Elements	% Parent Involvement	Primary Outcome Measures	Results	Effect Size
Piacentini et al,[19] 2011	71	12.2 y (8–17 y)	RCT (70:30): family CBT vs PRT	Parents attended full sessions 1 and 2, final 30 min of remaining: PE, contingency management, disengage from OCD behaviors, developmentally appropriate FI, relapse prevention, ERP	~50	• CGI-I (responder:<3) • CY-BOCS • COIS-R • FAS	• ITT analysis: FCBT 57.1% vs PRT 27.3% • Completer: FCBT 68.3% vs PRT 35.3% • FCBT 46.2% reduction, PRT 32% reduction (n.s. but effect size d = 0.40) • FCBT greater in reducing severity, child functional status; marginally significant for greater reduction in family accommodation of sx • FAS declined for FCBT, not PRT (d = 0.42) ◦ Reduced accommodation temporally preceded CY-BOCS improvement	FCBT: 2.37 (CYBOCS); 0.81 (COIS-RC); 1.01 (COIS-RP); 0.78 (FAS)

Study	n	Age	Design	Treatment components	%	Measures	Findings	Effect size
Reynolds et al,[20] 2013	50	14.5 y (12–17 y)	Randomized comparison: individual CBT vs parent-enhanced CBT	PE, accommodation, building hierarchy, behavioral experiments, rewarding progress	Individual CBT ~21 PE-CBT: 100	• CY-BOCS (response≤14)	• Individual CBT 44%, PE-CBT: 48%, difference n.s. ○ Both high- and low-parental involvement effective ○ Parent-enhanced CBT may be associated with significantly larger reductions in anxiety	1.45 I-CBT 1.27 PE-CBT
(POTS Jr) Freeman et al,[18] 2014	127	7.2 y (5–8 y)	RCT: FB-CBT vs FB-RT	PE, parent training, ERP, family treatment	100	• CY-BOCS • CGI-I • COIS-R	• FB-CBT superior to FB-RT, d = 0.84 • FB-CBT (72% responders) superior to FB-RT (41% responders), d = 0.31 • FB-CBT superior to FB-RT, d = 0.42	0.84 FB-CBT
Lewin et al,[21] 2014	31	5.8 y (3–8 y)	RCT: FB-ERP vs TAU	PE, parent tools (reduce accommodation, rewards, modeling), ERP, relapse and treatment maintenance	100	• CGI-I (responders much or very much improved) • CGI-S (remission≤mild) • CY-BOCS (% reduction) • CY-BOCS (remission≤12)	• FB-ERP 65%, TAU 7% • FB-ERP 35.2%, TAU 0% • FB-ERP 59% reduction, TAU 3% increase • FB-ERP 59%, TAU 0%	1.69 in favor of FB-ERP

+ Post-treatment effect size calculations: Within group treatment effect size was calculated based on means, standard deviations for those studies without reported effect sizes; studies were required to have at least 10 subjects for calculation. A weighted average of effect size and n were utilized for Barrett et al., 2004 and follow up studies given two family treatment groups.

Abbreviations: ADIS, anxiety disorders interview schedule; CBFT, cognitive-behavioral family therapy; CGI, clinical global impression; CGI-I, clinical global impression–improvement; CGI-S, clinical global impression-severity; COIS, child OCD impact scale; COIS-C, child OCD impact scale-child report; COIS-RC, child OCD impact scale revised-child report; COIS-RP, child OCD impact scale revised-parent report; CY-BOCS, children's Yale-Brown obsessive compulsive scale; ERP, exposure and response prevention; FAS, family accommodation scale; FB-CBT, family-based cognitive-behavioral therapy; FB-RT, family based relaxation treatment; FCBT, family CBT; FI, family involvement; ITT, intent to treat; M-FAD, McMaster family assessment device; NIMH GOCS, National Institute of Mental Health Global Obsessive Compulsive Scale; PE, psychoeducation; PFIT, positive family interaction therapy; POTS, pediatric obsessive-compulsive disorder treatment study; PRT, psychoeducation-relaxation training; RCT, randomized controlled trial; ST, standard treatment of individual CBT; TAU, treatment as usual.

Family accommodation is linked to OCD severity as well as treatment outcomes. Higher levels of family accommodation mediate the relationship between the severity of symptoms and parent-rated functional impairment.[25] Additionally, those children with higher baseline levels of family accommodation tend to fare worse across treatments[27] even when controlling for baseline severity.[28] Adjunctive family-based treatment aimed specifically to reduce family accommodation has recently been shown to improve and accelerate treatment response in adults,[29] highlighting accommodation as an important intervention target.

Family functioning

Because children exist within the context of the family system, how family members interact with each other in the presence of stressors is an important consideration when treating pediatric OCD. For example, OCD youth in families that have an antagonistic response style[30] or respond with critical comments and rejection[28] typically exhibit more severe symptoms and lower overall functioning. Families with higher conflict also have more difficulty disengaging from OCD rituals and accommodation patterns.[26] Higher levels of family dysfunction have also been linked to both poorer treatment response[31,32] and worse long-term outcomes.[11]

In families with a child with OCD, or anxiety in general, parent–child interactions tend to be characterized by lower overall warmth than nonanxious parent–child dyads. Parents of children with OCD tend to display less confidence in their child's abilities, engage in less positive problem solving, and are less likely to promote independence.[33] Parents of anxious youth globally tend to intervene and retain control over problem-solving tasks[34] and provide more limited opportunities for child-directed control.[35]

Family history and psychopathology

Parents of children who are anxious tend to also have a history of anxiety. Remarkably, youth of an anxious parent are between 5 to 7 times more likely to have an anxiety disorder than children of nonanxious parents.[36,37] Furthermore, family history of OCD is linked to smaller effect sizes across treatment modalities as well as dramatic attenuation of cognitive-behavioral therapy (CBT) response unless augmented with medication.[27] Parents with a history of OCD may have an especially difficult time disengaging from accommodation or engaging in exposure and response prevention (ERP).

Empirical Support for Family-Based Intervention in Pediatric Obsessive-Compulsive Disorder

At present, CBT including ERP as a monotherapy or in combination with serotonin reuptake inhibitors (SRIs) is considered to be the superior treatment approach[38] and yields a large pooled effect size across clinical trials.[39] However, given that half the children and adolescents with OCD do not respond to ERP alone,[38,40] ways to improve treatment outcomes are needed.

A recent meta-analysis investigated the overall effect of family inclusive treatment (FIT) on outcomes in OCD.[22] Based on 29 studies, FIT had a large effect on both symptom reduction and functioning, across a wide range of formats and level of family involvement. Importantly, the sole moderator of treatment impact on symptom reduction was the number of family-based sessions, with more sessions related to more favorable outcomes.

Initial open-label studies showed that family-based treatment could be successfully implemented and obtain significant reductions in symptoms and family accommodation, regardless of durational format (weekly vs intensive; see **Table 1**). More recently,

5 randomized controlled trials (RCTs) involving family-based CBT (FB-CBT) indicate large effects on symptom reduction and functional improvement in youth with OCD when compared with community-based treatment, including a study demonstrating robust changes 7 years after treatment (see **Table 1**).

Family-based approaches tend to converge on several common treatment elements. These include provision of psychoeducation to the parents and child, orientation to parent skills (eg, tolerance of personal distress, differential attention, modeling, scaffolding the child's autonomy when engaging in skills), problem solving, establishing effective reward systems, addressing family process elements that disrupt therapeutic progress (eg, family accommodation, parental negativity, family communication), and discussion of relapse prevention.[41] See later discussion in the context of clinical application.

Positive family interaction therapy (PFIT) is another form of family-based treatment that has been evaluated as an adjunct to individual child CBT. PFIT emphasizes skills that address family-level dynamics and processes known to interfere with OCD treatment response.[42] In a preliminary trial, families with high levels of blame, conflict, and poor cohesion were randomized to receive either standard individual CBT or CBT plus 6 sessions of PFIT.[42] Although both groups evidenced symptom improvement, a weighted mean effect size difference of 0.65 favored the PFIT condition. This study highlights that, in complicated cases of pediatric OCD with high levels of family dysfunction, targeted family-based interventions are superior to CBT with standard of care elements (eg, ERP).

The authors' FB-CBT approach is described below in detail, including evaluation procedures, treatment goals, and therapeutic intervention techniques.[18] This treatment integrates elements of biological, developmental, learning, and family dynamic models.[10,14] In addition, involving additional therapeutic techniques from other empirically-based treatments (eg, mindfulness-based strategies, motivational interviewing) can be beneficial in promoting treatment engagement. The authors' FB-CBT approach is described below in detail, including evaluation procedures, treatment goals, and therapeutic intervention techniques.

PATIENT EVALUATION OVERVIEW

Treatment of OCD begins with a thorough assessment of symptoms, degree of interference, and functional impairment. In the case of children and adolescents, evaluation of family-level factors (eg, accommodation, family distress, communications skills) is also essential. Generally speaking, the authors use the Children's Yale-Brown Obsessive Compulsive Scale (CY-BOCS) and the Anxiety Disorders Interview Schedule (ADIS) to assess OCD symptoms and comorbid diagnoses. However, we commonly use several additional assessment tools to screen for comorbidity rule-outs, gather additional information about functional impairment, and further assess family dynamics (**Table 2**).

The assessment process focuses on whether symptoms are developmentally normative and on the level of involvement of parents, siblings, teachers, and friends in OCD behaviors. Furthermore, a careful understanding of the child's core fears and family accommodation will help pinpoint key considerations for treatment (eg, particular exposure targets, needed family communication skills).

TREATMENT GOALS

Treatment of OCD includes several goals that facilitate improvement in symptoms and functioning, including reduction of family accommodation of OCD, enhancing

Table 2 Typical obsessive-compulsive disorder assessment measures	
Measure	**Description**
Children's Yale-Brown Obsessive Compulsive Scale (CY-BOCS)	Semistructured assessment of symptoms, severity
Family Accommodation Scale (FAS)	13-item questionnaire of family involvement in OCD rituals
Child OCD Impact Scale (COIS)	56-item self- or parent-report of functional impact of OCD across psychosocial domains
Anxiety Disorders Interview Schedule for Children (ADIS-C)	Structured assessment of DSM-IV childhood anxiety and comorbid disorders
Multidimensional Anxiety Scale for Children (MASC)	39-item self-report of anxiety symptoms
Children's Depression Inventory (CDI)	27-item self-report of depressive symptoms
Additional Measures	
Family Assessment Measure III (FAM-III)	50-item self-report of family relationships and interactions
Kiddie Schedule for Affective Disorders and Schizophrenia for school-aged children: Present and Lifetime (K-SADS-P/L)	Semistructured assessment across range of DSM-IV criteria, particularly useful for autism-spectrum disorders
Yale Global Tic Severity Scale (YGTSS)	Semistructured assessment of motor/vocal tics, severity

Abbreviation: DSM-IV, Diagnostic and Statistical Manual of Mental Disorders, Fourth Edition.
Adapted from Sapyta JJ, Freeman J, Franklin ME, et al. Obsessive compulsive disorder. Cognitive-behavior therapy for children and adolescents. Washington, DC: American Psychiatric Publishing; 2012. p. 305.

tolerance to OCD triggers via ERP, and increased flexibility through learning and implementing new coping strategies. Furthermore, family support of the overall treatment model is integral, ranging from a role as a cotherapist in the case of younger children, to helping initiate and carry out ERP tasks, to increasing functional family communication skills. Additionally, parents play a critical role in either helping or hindering treatment compliance, including medication and between-session practice of therapeutic skills.

CLINICAL APPLICATION: FAMILY-BASED COGNITIVE-BEHAVIORAL THERAPY

The current treatment protocol was developed for family-based treatment of early-emerging OCD[18] and is rooted in the well-established treatment developed for treatment of pediatric OCD.[14] Although originally implemented with young children, this treatment program is easily adapted for use with older children and adolescents.

The treatment protocol is typically 12 to 14 sessions delivered weekly. The format of the treatment program progresses as follows: (1) psychoeducation, (2) behavior management skills training (parent tools), (3) externalizing OCD and graded ERP (child tools), and (4) family process issues; summarized in **Table 3**.

Psychoeducation for Parents

As with most individual CBT treatments of OCD, this treatment program begins with psychoeducation about OCD. With young children, this is first accomplished with parents alone during 2 initial 90-minute sessions to introduce key points. This is contrasted with individual treatment models or family-based models with older children

Table 3
Family-based cognitive-behavioral therapy treatment summary

Family-Based CBT Component Summary	
Psychoeducation	• OCD in neurobehavioral framework • Treatment rationale • Normative rituals vs OCD • Psychoeducation tailored to youth's developmental level
Parent Tools	• Differential attention • Modeling • Scaffolding
Child Tools	• Externalizing OCD • Fear thermometer • ERP
Family Processes	• Reduction of accommodation • Family problem solving • Enhanced communication skills

and adolescents, in which psychoeducation is often provided in initial sessions with both the parent and child together.[12,14] Parents are introduced to the neurobiological framework of OCD and misattributions about OCD are amended. Functionally, this helps alleviate blame and introduces optimism about the treatment of OCD. Families are provided with information about recent advances in the treatment of OCD to instill hope; however, they are also given the place to process sadness, fear, and resentment about the impact of OCD on their child's and their family's functioning.

At this stage, it is also important to discuss normative obsessive-compulsive behavior (eg, annoying song that gets stuck in one's head, rigidity in routines in early childhood) and differentiate that from OCD behaviors that additionally are intrusive and ego-dystonic. This is emphasized to help parents distinguish between OCD and non-OCD behaviors and identify ways in which OCD causes problems for their child and family (**Table 4**).

The clinician then aims to clarify typical patterns observed in OCD, how families become intricately involved in OCD rituals, and how family-based treatment can begin to help alleviate symptoms and distress. It is critical for parents to understand clearly the treatment rationale, as well as the overall agenda of the treatment program. Key ideas to establish early with parents include discussion that they too will endure distress as they observe their child experience anxiety, that treatment will likely seek to alter current family routines and practices, and that dedication to between-session practice is essential for improvement. Parents thus gain an understanding of their role in treatment as active participants who critically promote behavioral change.

CLINICAL VIGNETTE: FAMILY ACCOMMODATION OBSERVED WITH YOUNG CHILD

Presentation: Eva is a 6-year old girl who has become increasingly concerned with germs. Her parents describe how Eva will visually check toys and eating utensils for spots or blemishes and will ask repeatedly if everyday objects are clean enough to use. When she finds spots on objects, she will ask her parents to clean them for her. Until recently, they have been obliging her requests, particularly during transitions, but it has become increasingly worse. She has begun to refuse to touch anything her siblings have used and becomes very upset when her younger brother touches her toys. Her parents indicate that during the past 2 weeks at school, Eva's teacher has seen her stand near her desk instead of sit down, use hand sanitizer frequently, spend more time in the bathroom, and she is even starting to avoid playtime activities with friends.

- *Evaluation: Full developmental history to rule out neurologic, developmental issue, comorbidity (eg, tics, disruptive behavior, generalized anxiety). Explicitly obtain full history of symptoms and parents' understanding of Eva's fears, behaviors, and rituals.*
  - *ADIS*
  - *CY-BOCS*
- *Family accommodation: As part of the intake, clinician should gain a full understanding of accommodation. How do parents respond to requests to clean? Do they offer reassurance? What happens to Eva's anxiety if they do so or not? What happens when she refuses to touch items handled by her siblings? How are family routines affected by Eva's fears? What about at school?*
  - *Family Accommodation Scale (FAS) as needed*
- *Plan: Contextualize these behaviors as OCD, a hiccough in Eva's brain that makes her focus more on germs, begin psychoeducation about OCD, treatment, and family involvement in OCD rituals.*

Psychoeducation for Children

Beginning in the third session with younger children, psychoeducation is provided to the child in a developmentally appropriate manner, making ample use of metaphors, imagery, and examples. A special goal of psychoeducation with the child (and parents) is to externalize OCD as separate from the child (eg, giving OCD a nickname or simply labeling as OCD). Psychoeducation with the child should portray OCD as an entity that intends to undermine the child's true wishes (like a bully or annoying younger sibling), as well as introduce the idea that the child can be the boss of OCD behaviors. Facilitating the child's understanding of how OCD works is critical for next steps in providing the rationale for ERP and identifying ways to reduce ways that OCD "bosses" or "bullies" the child.

Table 4 Developmentally appropriate rituals and fears found in children	
Age	**Normal Behavioral Rigidity and Rituals**
1–2	Strong preference for rigid around-home routines (eg, nighttime, bath time). Very aware and can get upset about imperfections in toys or clothes.
3–5	Play activities are repeated over and over (and over) again.
5–6	Keen awareness of the rules of games and other activities (eg, classroom rules) and may become upset if rules are altered or broken.
6–11	Engage in superstitious behavior to prevent bad things from happening (eg, do not step on a crack). May show increased interest in acquiring a collection of objects.
12+	Become easily absorbed in particular enjoyable activities (eg, video games) or with particular people (eg, pop stars, athletes). May show superstitious behavior in relation to making good things happen (eg, performance in sports).

Data from Freeman JB, Garcia AM. Family based treatment for young children with OCD: therapist guide. New York: Oxford University Press; 2008; and Evans DW, Leckman JF, Carter A, et al. Ritual, habit, and perfectionism: the prevalence and development of compulsive-like behaviour in normal young children. Child Dev 1997;68(1):58–68.

Parent Tools

To ensure sustainability of interventions and facilitate between-session practice of therapeutic skills, parents are trained as coaches or cotherapists for their children. This enables families to support effective use of ERP outside of the therapy room while extricating themselves from OCD rituals.

Differential Attention

To help caregivers manage distress associated with OCD treatment, the authors have integrated parent-training elements into the FB-CBT protocol, including increased positive attention, planned ignoring, and use of a reward program.[43,44] Parents are encouraged to target positive non-OCD behaviors with appropriate prompts and praise. Parents also learn how to disengage from OCD behavior with planned ignoring, including engaging in less eye contact, verbal interaction, and touch. Older children may be more interested in increased autonomy and privileges, and these can take the place of prizes or special time with parents.

Modeling

Parents are encouraged to monitor how escalations in their own distress influence how the child interacts with OCD. Thus, as they become more skilled in coping and ERP strategies, parents can model adaptive responses to OCD behaviors.

It is also important to note the parallel modeling process of therapist to parents. It can be beneficial for families to see how the clinician responds to OCD symptoms and encourages the child to use skills in session. By learning how the clinician interacts with the child's OCD symptoms, parents learn how to implement ERP, monitor symptoms, map current OCD behaviors, and broaden their response repertoire to reassurance seeking and other OCD symptoms.

Scaffolding

Just as therapists aim to increase parent and child tolerance of anxiety and independent use of tools, parents also are tasked with helping the child increasingly manage distress independently. To achieve this, parents encourage the child to increase use of coping tools and scale back their own efforts to step in and directly alleviate child distress. However, watching one's child in distress is distressing! Helping parents learn how to manage their own anxiety is integral to helping children manage theirs.

Child or Adolescent Tools

Externalizing obsessive-compulsive disorder

The first child tool emphasized in treatment is externalization of OCD. This begins during psychoeducation, when the clinician models with externalizing language and encourages the child to separate OCD processes from the self by naming them with either an irreverent nickname (eg, Booger Man) or labeling simply as OCD. The authors encourage clinicians to draw on the child and family's creativity. With young children, it may be helpful to have the child draw a picture of OCD or develop an OCD character.

Fear thermometer

The fear thermometer is used to rate and monitor the child's subjective anxiety level. The clinician frequently checks in with the child (and parents), asking them to rate their anxiety level according to a developmentally appropriate rating scale (eg, analog visual faces scale with small child, 1–10 with adolescent). Ultimately, the fear thermometer provides a tool for the child to report distress efficiently.

Exposure and response prevention with family disengagement from obsessive-compulsive disorder

ERP in the context of FB-CBT aims to increase the family's ability to manage the feared situations (with the appropriate coping tools in hand) rather than avoid or escape them.

ERP progresses in much the same ways as outlined in individual CBT treatment, with one significant difference: parents are involved directly with exposure tasks. Exposures at first will be conducted by the therapist with the parent observing. Then, the therapist will scaffold transfer of exposure tasks to the parent over time. Additionally, when conducting exposures, parents will practice tolerating their own anxiety and modeling adaptive behavioral responses to OCD.

Family dynamics

Understanding the contextual and family processes is critical to successful implementation of this family-based treatment program. Accommodation of OCD is typically an instinctive practice because it serves to alleviate child and parent distress as well as keep the family functioning. Thus, helping parents be more mindful of how they habitually interact with the child's symptoms of OCD is crucial for success.

Changing the ways in which families interact with OCD may lead to arguments and challenges to family functioning. As a result, it is critical to help the family increase positive communication and problem-solving skills. The authors have found it beneficial to help families identify predictable patterns of behavior related to worsening of symptoms and subsequent disruptions in family functioning. Coaching communication skills, such as active listening, labeling personal feelings or thoughts with "I think" or "I feel" statements, establishing ground rules for when to discuss tough topics, and identifying common communication traps, can improve family discourse and make emotional conversations more connecting.

COMBINATION OR PHARMACOLOGIC THERAPIES

Although CBT is the standard first-line treatment of mild-to-moderate OCD, the most recent American Academy of Child and Adolescent Psychiatry (AACAP) standards designate that in moderate-to-severe cases medication is indicated in combination with CBT.[45] Current empirical data indicate SRIs as first-line medication to be implemented in combination with CBT for the treatment of pediatric OCD.[45] As observed in the Pediatric Obsessive-Compulsive Disorder Treatment Study (POTS) trial, effect sizes for combination therapy tend to reflect the additive effects of CBT and medication monotherapies (ie, 1.4, 0.97, 0.67, respectively).[38] A 2003 meta-analysis comparing the effects of SRIs in RCTs indicated a combined pooled effect size of 0.46, significantly greater than placebo, with clomipramine significantly greater than selective SRIs (SSRIs; eg, fluoxetine, sertraline, fluvoxamine, paroxetine, citalopram), which were equally superior to placebo.[46] Despite this, SSRIs tend to be the first choice for children given common adverse effects of clomipramine and necessary cardiac monitoring.[2,45]

The evidence cannot currently answer which SRI is best for which child, and current practice parameters reflect this evidentiary gap.[45] However, medication should generally be considered in moderate-to-severe cases, including CY-BOCS scores at or above 23 or if functional impairment is marked.[45] The original POTS trial found that in children with a first-degree relative with OCD, CBT was 6 times more effective when an SRI medication was also a part of the treatment.[27] Those children who present with comorbid tics are likely to fare better with CBT or CBT combined with medication but not medication alone.[47]

Monitoring the child's response to medication closely to attain the highest tolerated dose will result in more positive outcomes. This is accomplished more frequently by involving the family in the monitoring process and addressing any symptoms that directly interfere with adherence.

TREATMENT RESISTANCE

The empirical literature suggests that for some children, a time-limited course of CBT treatment is not entirely effective. Indeed, as many as one-third to one-half of children with OCD could be considered treatment-resistant, meaning they do not fully benefit from established efficacious treatments.[45] In these cases, the authors suggest that family-based treatment is especially helpful because as symptoms and level of functional impairment increase so does the likelihood of problematic family factors (eg, parent–child interaction style, parental negativity, family accommodation). However, the evidence for FB-CBT is also just emerging and marked by nonresponders to treatment. Thus, in cases of nonresponse or partial response, extension of treatment is warranted, including (1) medication augmentation, (2) further involvement of family members in treatment and alternative family-based approaches (eg, emerging evidence for PFIT, previously described[42]; FB-CBT in response to medication nonresponse),[48] or (3) increased intensity of treatment (eg, longer duration, more frequent sessions).

CLINICAL VIGNETTE: IDENTITY CONTAGION AND TREATMENT RESISTANCE

Presentation: Marissa is a 13-year-old girl who has been receiving individual CBT treatment of OCD for more than 2 years. She is currently on her second trial of an SSRI. Her symptoms have persisted despite a recent increase, albeit she is not yet at the maximum tolerated dose. Her obsessions have recently involved contagion thinking and scrupulosity. Specifically, she expresses concerns of being blasphemous because she started working on a school project with a classmate who identifies as atheist. She believes her classmate is likable and kind but she also has intrusive thoughts that if she accepts her classmate's ideas into her project her own beliefs on spirituality could be tainted. Marissa also expresses concerns that she could be responsible for her damnation if she does not pray perfectly every night. Her compulsive praying includes striving for an experience of "an open heart and visualizing a smiling Jesus," otherwise she might be praying to Satan. During a recent session, she noted that she has begun to feel disconnected from her family and her church. She repeatedly talks to her parents and her youth pastor questioning if her faith is sincere and they have reassured repeatedly that her acute concern is evidence that her heart is in the right place.

- *Plan: Obsessions based on spirituality need to be treated with the utmost sensitivity and with frequent family processing and involvement. Because of Marissa's family's devout religious background, it is important to involve them in discussion and planning of exposures related to her current fears, particularly with discussing appropriate exposure targets (ie, explicitly only ones that she is "stuck" thinking about).*

- *Involving the family, OCD should be framed as exploiting Marissa's spiritual values and the family's desire to help. Family members can both model appropriate adherence to the family's faith and encourage exposure targets that are clear, acceptable externalizations of the family's faith.*

- *Given Marissa's symptom recurrence and severe presentation, additional consultation with her child psychiatrist is warranted. Because she is experiencing persistent symptoms, she should continue with a medication increase to the maximum tolerated dose consistent with positive response or to the point at which adverse event (eg, side effect) is experienced.*

The most common medication augmentation strategy is adding clomipramine to the child's current SSRI, thereby enhancing serotonergic effects.[45] No RCTs have evaluated the effects of medication augmentation with atypical neuroleptics in children; however, preliminary evidence supports that after 2 or more failed trials of SSRIs or enhancement with clomipramine, atypical neuroleptics may be considered.

EVALUATION OF OUTCOME AND LONG-TERM RECOMMENDATIONS

Evaluation of symptoms and functional status should be an ongoing process occurring throughout treatment. Typically, treatment-outcomes are evaluated based on both short-term and long-term goals set with the family.

As the child and family begin to achieve treatment goals of reduced compulsive behavior and reduced family accommodation, and as functional status is improved, the clinician and family need to prepare for longer term goals beyond therapy. The clinician may revisit psychoeducational conversations that addressed the waxing-and-waning nature of OCD, review progress, and highlight tools that the family and child now have that prepare them to (1) predict and identify the reappearance of OCD symptoms and (2) to face such future OCD symptoms with demonstrated bravery, creativity, and family support to mediate a symptom flare from turning into full relapse.

Indeed, because OCD symptoms tend to wax and wane, treatment response can be conceptualized and talked about with families as "living with Os and Cs." Even though obsessions might emerge again, the child and family have learned how to interact with it in such a way (ie, not engaging in compulsions) that the experience of obsessions is short-lived and not interfering; in other words, removing the "D" from the equation.

SUMMARY

There is growing consensus that CBT approaches for pediatric OCD must include substantial family-based elements to improve treatment compliance and address functional family accommodation. Effective family-based treatment identifies and addresses family dynamics that affect the development and maintenance of OCD symptoms. Simultaneously, family members learn to manage anxiety associated with OCD and develop tools that increase their adaptive coping skills. Increased research will continue to strengthen ongoing clinical implementation of family-based treatment. Ultimately, these efforts will improve outcomes for children with OCD and their families.

REFERENCES

1. Angst J, Gamma A, Endrass J, et al. Obsessive-compulsive severity spectrum in the community: prevalence, comorbidity, and course. Eur Arch Psychiatry Clin Neurosci 2004;254(3):156–64.
2. Flament MF, Whitaker A, Rapoport JL, et al. Obsessive compulsive disorder in adolescence: an epidemiological study. J Am Acad Child Adolesc Psychiatry 1988;27(6):764–71.
3. Rapoport JL, Inoff-Germain G, Weissman MM, et al. Childhood obsessive-compulsive disorder in the NIMH MECA study: parent versus child identification of cases. J Anxiety Disord 2000;14(6):535–48.
4. Zohar AH. The epidemiology of obsessive-compulsive disorder in children and adolescents. Child Adolesc Psychiatr Clin N Am 1999;8(3):445–60.

5. Piacentini J, Bergman RL, Keller M, et al. Functional impairment in children and adolescents with obsessive-compulsive disorder. J Child Adolesc Psychopharmacol 2003;13(2, Supplement 1):61–9.

6. Piacentini J, Jaffer M. Measuring functional impairment in youngsters with OCD: manual for the child OCD Impact Scale (COIS). Los Angeles (CA): UCLA Department of Psychiatry; 1999.

7. Farrell LJ, Barrett PM. The function of the family in childhood obsessive-compulsive disorder: family interactions and accommodation. In: Storch EA, Geffken GR, Murphy TK, editors. Handbook of child and adolescent obsessive-compulsive disorder. Mahwah, NJ: Lawrence Erlbaum Associates, Inc; 2007. p. 313–32.

8. Waters TL, Barrett PM, March JS. Cognitive-behavioral family treatment of childhood obsessive-compulsive disorder: preliminary findings. Am J Psychother 2001;55(3):372–87.

9. Grunes MS, Neziroglu F, McKay D. Family involvement in the behavioral treatment of obsessive-compulsive disorder: a preliminary investigation. Behav Ther 2001; 32(4):803–20.

10. Freeman JB, Garcia AM, Fucci C, et al. Family-based treatment of early-onset obsessive-compulsive disorder. J Child Adolesc Psychopharmacol 2003;13(2, Supplement 1):71–80.

11. Barrett P, Farrell L, Dadds M, et al. Cognitive-behavioral family treatment of childhood obsessive-compulsive disorder: long-term follow-up and predictors of outcome. J Am Acad Child Adolesc Psychiatry 2005;44(10):1005–14.

12. Barrett P, Healy-Farrell L, March JS. Cognitive-behavioral family treatment of childhood obsessive-compulsive disorder: a controlled trial. J Am Acad Child Adolesc Psychiatry 2004;43(1):46–62.

13. Martin J, Thienemann M. Group cognitive-behavior therapy with family involvement for middle-school-age children with obsessive-compulsive disorder: a pilot study. Child Psychiatry Hum Dev 2005;36(1):113–27.

14. March JS, Mulle K. OCD in children and adolescents: a cognitive-behavioral treatment manual. New York: Guilford Press; 1998.

15. Storch EA, Geffken GR, Merlo LJ, et al. Family-based cognitive-behavioral therapy for pediatric obsessive-compulsive disorder: comparison of intensive and weekly approaches. J Am Acad Child Adolesc Psychiatry 2007;46(4):469–78.

16. Freeman JB, Garcia AM, Coyne L, et al. Early childhood OCD: preliminary findings from a family-based cognitive-behavioral approach. J Am Acad Child Adolesc Psychiatry 2008;47(5):593–602.

17. O'Leary EM, Barrett P, Fjermestad KW. Cognitive-behavioral family treatment for childhood obsessive-compulsive disorder: a 7-year follow-up study. J Anxiety Disord 2009;23(7):973–8.

18. Freeman J, Sapyta J, Garcia A, et al. Family-based treatment of early childhood obsessive-compulsive disorder: the Pediatric Obsessive-Compulsive Disorder Treatment Study for Young Children (POTS Jr)—a randomized clinical trial. JAMA psychiatry 2014;71(6):689–98.

19. Piacentini J, Bergman RL, Chang S, et al. Controlled comparison of family cognitive behavioral therapy and psychoeducation/relaxation training for child obsessive-compulsive disorder. J Am Acad Child Adolesc Psychiatry 2011; 50(11):1149–61.

20. Reynolds SA, Clark S, Smith H, et al. Randomized controlled trial of parent-enhanced CBT compared with individual CBT for obsessive-compulsive disorder in young people. J Consult Clin Psychol 2013;81(6):1021.

21. Lewin AB, Park JM, Jones AM, et al. Family-based exposure and response prevention therapy for preschool-aged children with obsessive-compulsive disorder: a pilot randomized controlled trial. Behav Res Ther 2014;56:30–8.

22. Thompson-Hollands J, Edson A, Tompson MC, et al. Family involvement in the psychological treatment of obsessive-compulsive disorder: a meta-analysis. J Fam Psychol 2014;28(3):287–98.

23. Stewart SE, Beresin C, Haddad S, et al. Predictors of family accommodation in obsessive-compulsive disorder. Ann Clin Psychiatry 2008;20(2):65–70.

24. Stewart SE, Hu YP, Hezel DM, et al. Development and psychometric properties of the OCD Family Functioning (OFF) scale. J Fam Psychol 2011;25(3):434.

25. Storch EA, Geffken GR, Merlo LJ, et al. Family accommodation in pediatric obsessive-compulsive disorder. J Clin Child Adolesc Psychol 2007;36(2):207–16.

26. Peris TS, Bergman RL, Langley A, et al. Correlates of accommodation of pediatric obsessive-compulsive disorder: parent, child, and family characteristics. J Am Acad Child Adolesc Psychiatry 2008;47(10):1173–81.

27. Garcia AM, Sapyta JJ, Moore PS, et al. Predictors and moderators of treatment outcome in the Pediatric Obsessive Compulsive Treatment Study (POTS I). J Am Acad Child Adolesc Psychiatry 2010;49(10):1024–33.

28. Amir N, Freshman M, Foa EB. Family distress and involvement in relatives of obsessive-compulsive disorder patients. J Anxiety Disord 2000;14(3):209–17.

29. Thompson-Hollands J, Abramovitch A, Tompson MC, et al. A randomized clinical trial of a brief family intervention to reduce accommodation in obsessive-compulsive disorder: a preliminary study. Behav Ther 2015;46(2):218–29.

30. Renshaw KD, Steketee G, Chambless DL. Involving family members in the treatment of OCD. Cogn Behav Ther 2005;34(3):164–75.

31. Barrett P, Dadds M, Rapee RM. Family treatment of childhood anxiety: a controlled trial. J Consult Clin Psychol 1996;64(2):333.

32. Peris TS, Sugar CA, Bergman RL, et al. Family factors predict treatment outcome for pediatric obsessive-compulsive disorder. J Consult Clin Psychol 2012;80(2):255.

33. Barrett P, Shortt A, Healy L. Do parent and child behaviours differentiate families whose children have obsessive-compulsive disorder from other clinic and non-clinic families? J Child Psychol Psychiatry 2002;43(5):597–607.

34. Krohne HW, Hock M. Relationships between restrictive mother-child interactions and anxiety of the child. Anxiety Res 1991;4(2):109–24.

35. Chorpita BF, Brown TA, Barlow DH. Perceived control as a mediator of family environment in etiological models of childhood anxiety. Behav Ther 1998;29(3):457–76.

36. Beidel DC, Turner SM. At risk for anxiety: I. Psychopathology in the offspring of anxious parents. J Am Acad Child Adolesc Psychiatry 1997;36(7):918–24.

37. Turner SM, Beidel DC, Costello A. Psychopathology in the offspring of anxiety disorders patients. J Consult Clin Psychol 1987;55(2):229.

38. Pediatric OCD Treatment Study (POTS) Team. Cognitive-behavior therapy, sertraline, and their combination for children and adolescents with obsessive-compulsive disorder: the Pediatric OCD Treatment Study (POTS) randomized controlled trial. JAMA 2004;292(16):1969–76.

39. Watson HJ, Rees CS. Meta-analysis of randomized, controlled treatment trials for pediatric obsessive-compulsive disorder. J Child Psychol Psychiatry 2008;49(5):489–98.

40. Ginsburg GS, Kingery JN, Drake KL, et al. Predictors of treatment response in pediatric obsessive-compulsive disorder. J Am Acad Child Adolesc Psychiatry 2008;47(8):868–78.

41. Drake KL, Ginsburg GS. Family factors in the development, treatment, and prevention of childhood anxiety disorders. Clin Child Fam Psychol Rev 2012; 15(2):144–62.
42. Peris TS, Piacentini J. Optimizing treatment for complex cases of childhood obsessive compulsive disorder: a preliminary trial. J Clin Child Adolesc Psychol 2013;42(1):1–8.
43. Forehand RL, McMahon RJ. Helping the noncompliant child: a clinician's guide to parent training. New York: Guilford press; 1981.
44. Kazdin AE. Parent management training: evidence, outcomes, and issues. J Am Acad Child Adolesc Psychiatry 1997;36(10):1349–56.
45. Geller DA, March J. Practice parameter for the assessment and treatment of children and adolescents with obsessive-compulsive disorder. J Am Acad Child Adolesc Psychiatry 2012;51(1):98–113.
46. Geller DA, Biederman J, Stewart SE, et al. Which SSRI? A meta-analysis of pharmacotherapy trials in pediatric obsessive-compulsive disorder. Am J Psychiatry 2003;160(11):1919–28.
47. March JS, Franklin ME, Leonard H, et al. Tics moderate treatment outcome with sertraline but not cognitive-behavior therapy in pediatric obsessive-compulsive disorder. Biol Psychiatry 2007;61(3):344–7.
48. Storch EA, Lehmkuhl HD, Ricketts E, et al. An open trial of intensive family based cognitive-behavioral therapy in youth with obsessive-compulsive disorder who are medication partial responders or nonresponders. J Clin Child Adolesc Psychol 2010;39(2):260–8.

Trauma-focused Cognitive Behavior Therapy for Traumatized Children and Families

Judith A. Cohen, MD*, Anthony P. Mannarino, PhD

KEYWORDS

- Children • Adolescents • Trauma • PTSD • Parents • Families
- Trauma-focused CBT • Treatment

KEY POINTS

- Trauma-focused cognitive behavioral therapy (TF-CBT) is a family-focused treatment in which parents or caregivers (hereafter referred to as "parents") participate equally with their traumatized child or adolescent (hereafter referred to as "child").
- TF-CBT is a components-based and phase-based treatment that emphasizes proportionality and incorporates gradual exposure into each component.
- Parents and child receive all TF-CBT components in parallel individual sessions that allow parents and child to express their personal thoughts and feelings about the child's trauma experiences, gain skills to help the child reregulate trauma responses, and master avoidance of trauma reminders and memories.
- Families also participate in several conjoint parent-child sessions to enhance family communication about the child's trauma experiences and parental support of the child.
- Research documents that parental participation significantly enhances the beneficial impact of TF-CBT for traumatized children.

OVERVIEW: NATURE OF THE PROBLEM

Child trauma is a serious societal problem. At least 1 trauma is reported by two-thirds of American children and adolescents (hereafter referred to as "children"); 33% of children experience multiple traumas before reaching adulthood.[1] Although most children are resilient, trauma exposure is associated with increased risk for medical and mental

Disclosures: Drs J. A. Cohen and A. P. Mannarino receive grant funding from NIMH (Grant No MH R01 95208) and SAMHSA (Grant No SM 061257) and book royalties from Guilford Press.
Department of Psychiatry, Allegheny General Hospital, Drexel University College of Medicine, 4 Allegheny Center, 8th Floor, Pittsburgh, PA 15212, USA
* Corresponding author.
E-mail address: Jcohen1@wpahs.org

Abbreviations

PTSD   Posttraumatic Stress Disorder
TF-CBT   Trauma-focused cognitive behavior therapy

health problems including posttraumatic stress disorder (PTSD), depression, anxiety, substance abuse, and attempted and completed suicide.[2,3] Early identification and treatment of traumatized children can prevent these potentially serious and long-term negative outcomes.

Parents can have a significant impact on children's trauma responses. For example, lower levels of parental distress about the child's trauma and greater parental support predict more positive outcomes after child trauma exposure, whereas greater parental PTSD symptoms predict more negative child outcomes.[4] Involving parents in the traumatized child's treatment can effectively address these factors and thus positively affect the child's outcome.

Nonoffending parents are typically children's primary source of safety, support, and guidance. (Note that trauma-focused cognitive behavior therapy [TF-CBT] does not include offending parents; ie, parents who perpetrated the trauma for which the child is receiving treatment, such as a parent who perpetrated the child's sexual abuse or domestic violence.) However, trauma experiences teach children that the world is dangerous and that adults may not protect them. Such children often become angry at and stop trusting their parents, leading parents to become confused and upset. Trauma-focused therapy can help parents recognize and respond appropriately to their children's trauma responses while setting appropriate behavioral limits. This approach enables parents to provide the traumatized child with ongoing opportunities to relearn (or learn for the first time) that people can be safe and trustworthy. Thus, there are many reasons to suggest that family-focused treatment that integrally includes parents significantly enhances outcomes for traumatized children.

CHILD EVALUATION OVERVIEW

Evaluating children after trauma exposure is complex and is described in detail elsewhere.[5] There are important differences between forensic and clinical evaluations, particularly after child abuse.[6] The following discussion pertains only to clinical evaluations. As with all child mental health evaluations, these evaluations should include multiple informants. At a minimum this includes interviewing the child and parent, but school reports, pediatric records, and/or other information should also be obtained as clinically indicated, and this often includes speaking to or reviewing records from the child's Child Protective Services case worker, juvenile justice parole officer, and/or past and current psychiatric treatment providers (eg, medication prescriber, in-home or wraparound services, residential treatment facility). If a forensic evaluation has been conducted by the local child advocacy center or a private evaluator, these records should also be reviewed and included in the evaluation.

To benefit from TF-CBT, children must have experienced at least 1 remembered trauma. The remembered trauma can be any type of trauma, including multiple traumas or complex trauma. Because avoidance is a hallmark of PTSD, children often initially minimize information about their trauma experiences and symptoms; in some cases they may completely deny having experienced trauma, thus contributing to underdiagnosis of trauma-related disorders. In addition, as noted earlier, trauma involves the betrayal of trust, typically by adults; meeting a new adult, such as a therapist, can therefore serve as a trauma reminder and lead to high levels of mistrust during the initial evaluation, particularly for children with early interpersonal trauma and attachment disruption (complex trauma).

Children should have prominent trauma-related symptoms. A PTSD diagnosis is not necessary, although some PTSD symptoms are typically present. The use of a validated screening instrument, such as the University of California, Los Angeles PTSD Reaction Index for Diagnostic and Statistical Manual of Mental Disorders, Fifth Edition[7] or the Children's Posttraumatic Symptom Scale,[8] may be useful for following these symptoms but is not a replacement for a thorough clinical interview. Evaluators must develop competence at interviewing children across the developmental spectrum for the range of trauma symptoms with which children may present. Other common diagnoses are depressive, anxiety, behavioral, or adjustment disorders. Therapists should clearly understand the manifestations of complex trauma and the multiple domains of trauma impact (ie, affective, behavioral, biological, cognitive, interpersonal, perceptual), rather than depending solely on diagnosis to determine appropriateness for trauma-focused treatment. At the same time, therapists must distinguish between complex trauma and other comorbidities. For example, children whose behavioral problems occur within a constellation of affective, biological, cognitive, and interpersonal dysregulation that is triggered by trauma reminders are likely to respond to TF-CBT, and must be differentiated from children with severe primary externalizing behavior problems (eg, conduct disorder) who are likely to benefit more from another evidence-based treatment that addresses these difficulties before embarking on trauma-focused treatment.

MANAGEMENT GOALS

As the description given earlier suggests, the goals of TF-CBT are to address and reregulate the individual child's domains of trauma impact, which may be summarized by, but are not limited to, the following:

(A) Affective, such as anxiety, sadness, anger, affective dysregulation

(B) Behavioral, such as avoidance of trauma reminders, self-injurious behaviors, maladaptive behaviors modeled during trauma (eg, sexual behaviors, bullying, aggression), noncompliance, severe behavioral dysregulation

(B) Biological, such as hypervigilance, poor sleep, increased startle, stomach aches, headaches, other somatic problems that interfere with functioning

(C) Cognitive/perceptual, such as intrusive trauma-related thoughts and memories, maladaptive trauma-related beliefs, dissociation, psychotic symptoms, cognitive dysregulation

(S) Social/school, such as impaired relationships with family, friends, peers; social withdrawal; decline in school concentration, performance, and/or attendance; impaired attachment and/or trust

DESCRIPTION OF TREATMENT
Core Trauma-focused Cognitive Behavior Therapy Principles

Core TF-CBT principles are (1) phase-based and components-based treatment, (2) component order and proportionality of phases, (3) the use of gradual exposure in TF-CBT, and (4) the importance of integrally including parents or other primary caregivers into TF-CBT treatment. The first 3 are briefly described here. More details about these principles are described on our free Web-based training site, TF-CBTWeb, available at www.musc.edu/tfcbt and elsewhere.[9,10] The remainder of this article addresses how parents are incorporated into TF-CBT treatment.

TF-CBT is a phase-based and components-based treatment, as shown in **Box 1**.

The 3 phases of TF-CBT are stabilization, trauma narration and processing, and integration and consolidation. The components of TF-CBT are summarized by the acronym PRACTICE: Psychoeducation, Parenting Skills, Relaxation Skills, Affect Modulation Skills, Cognitive Processing Skills, Trauma narrative and processing, In vivo mastery, Conjoint child-parent sessions; and Enhancing Safety and future development. These components are described in detail later.

Box 1
TF-CBT components and phases

Psychoeducation	Stabilization phase
Parenting skills	
Relaxation	
Affect modulation	
Cognitive processing	
Trauma narration and processing	Trauma narrative phase
In vivo mastery	Integration/consolidation phase
Conjoint child-parent sessions	
Enhancing safety (traumatic grief components; optional)	

Fidelity to the TF-CBT model is important to ensure positive outcomes. Fidelity to the TF-CBT model includes the following: (1) the PRACTICE components are provided in sequential order (with some flexibility within the stabilization skills as clinically indicated and addressing Enhancing Safety first when clinically appropriate); (2) all PRACTICE components are provided (with the exception of In Vivo Mastery when this is not clinically indicated), and (3) the 3 TF-CBT phases are provided in appropriate proportion and duration. For typical trauma treatment cases, TF-CBT duration is 12 to 15 sessions and each treatment phase receives about an equal number of treatment sessions (ie, 4–5 sessions/phase). For complex trauma cases, treatment duration is longer (16–25 sessions) and the proportionality is altered slightly with about half of the treatment (8–12 sessions) dedicated to stabilization skills and a quarter of the treatment (4–6 sessions) spent on trauma narrative and integration/consolidation phases, respectively, as described elsewhere.[11]

Gradual exposure is included in all of the TF-CBT components. During each session the therapist carefully calibrates and includes increasing exposure to trauma reminders while encouraging the child and parent to use skills learned in previous sessions in order to master the fear, anxiety, or other negative emotions evoked on exposure to these trauma memories. Through this process the child and parent learn new cognitions (eg, "I can talk about sexual abuse without crying"; "Maybe my child is not damaged by what happened"). With time and ongoing practice, these cognitions become stronger and generalize to other situations, gradually replacing the maladaptive ones they initially had about the child's traumatic experience. Current evidence suggests that this may be the underlying process through which trauma-related fear is diminished.[12]

Parental Involvement in Trauma-focused Cognitive Behavior Therapy

Parent involvement is an integral part of the TF-CBT model and parents receive as much time in the treatment as children. During most TF-CBT sessions, the therapist spends about 30 minutes individually with the child and 30 minutes individually with the parent. Conjoint child-parent sessions are included later in the TF-CBT model to optimize open children-parent communication, both generally and related to the child's trauma experiences, as described in detail later. This structure was selected rather than family sessions based on the rationale that child trauma significantly affects parents and children and thus both benefit from individual opportunities to process personal trauma responses before meeting together to do so.

The therapist meets with the parent each session to provide the parent with each PRACTICE component as the child is receiving that component. In this manner, the parent is able to help the child to practice using the appropriate TF-CBT skills during the week when the child is not in therapy. Many parents report that the TF-CBT skills are personally helpful to them, and that encouraging their children to use these is helpful in reminding the parent to use the skills as well. Often parents practice the skills together with their children at home and this encourages the development of family resilience rituals that continue long after the end of therapy. Another reason for individual parent sessions is to facilitate open therapist-parent communication about difficult topics. For example, parents may use demeaning language to describe the child's behaviors, use ineffective discipline strategies, or say hurtful things to the child about the trauma. In such situations individual parent sessions allow the therapist to provide more appropriate parenting skills, as described later.

Most children in foster care have experienced trauma. As described later, including foster parents in treatment can enhance engagement and treatment completion for these children. In these cases, the therapist can also include the birth parent in TF-CBT if the therapist considers this to be clinically appropriate (eg, if the child is having regular visits with this parent and/or reunification is anticipated in the near future). Typically the therapist sees the birth parent in individual sessions at a separate time from the child and foster parent, and provides the birth parent with the same information as the foster parent. If the visits with the birth parent are going well and both foster parent and birth parent desire this, the therapist may consider having some sessions that include the birth and foster parents together at some points during the treatment, if clinical judgment suggests that this would be beneficial. Whether or not the birth parent participates, it is important that whenever possible at least 1 consistent parenting figure participates with the child throughout the course of TF-CBT.

Orienting the Family to Trauma-focused Cognitive Behavior Therapy

From the beginning of treatment it is important for the therapist to help the family understand that TF-CBT is a collaborative child-parent, trauma-focused treatment. The therapist may find it useful to review the information from the child's assessment that led the therapist to conclude that trauma-focused treatment was appropriate. Collaborative child-parent treatment means that the child and parent both receive about equal time each session and that the treatment includes 2 way open communication about important issues. The parent and child may express discomfort about this (eg, lack of confidentiality in therapy). The therapist can often address this by asking each what their concerns are about sharing information and making appropriate adjustments to the extent to which this occurs when indicated. For example, youth with complex trauma who are attending TF-CBT with new foster parents often have understandable issues with trusting these new caregivers or even in trusting the therapist; the therapist needs to attend to this appropriately or the therapy may be derailed.[11]

The therapist also explains what trauma-focused treatment entails in TF-CBT; namely that (1) the therapist thinks that the following problems (the therapist specifies what these are here) are related to the child's trauma experiences; (2) these problems and their relationship to the child's trauma experiences are the focus of this treatment; and (3) this is the focus of TF-CBT and what the treatment will be addressing every session, even if other issues arise during the course of treatment. By clarifying the nature of trauma-focused treatment, the therapist helps the family to understand what to expect and also differentiates TF-CBT from other treatments (eg, usual care) that they may have received in the past.

We recognize that a variety of caregivers may participate in TF-CBT and in many cases these are not the child's legal parents and/or may be a single parent or caregiver. For consistency and simplicity, the term "parents" is used throughout the following description of TF-CBT components except where specifically noted.

STABILIZATION PHASE (4–12 SESSIONS)
Psychoeducation

During psychoeducation the therapist provides information about common trauma responses and trauma reminders, and connects these to the child's trauma experiences. The therapist also normalizes and validates these as trauma responses, because many children and parents view traumatic behavioral and affective dysregulation as the child having become a bad kid. Helping children and parents understand these as children's response to the bad things that have happened in their lives, and recognizing trauma reminders that may trigger these responses, is often extremely helpful in changing the child's and parent's perspective on the problem. Importantly, this gives them hope that the child can recover and return to more positive functioning, even if the child has a long history of complex trauma and long-standing dysregulation. As with all TF-CBT components, the therapist individually tailors how to provide psychoeducation, taking into consideration the developmental level, culture, and interests of the child and family. This approach may include playing interactive psychoeducational games such as the What Do You Know game,[13] or, for teens, discussing psychoeducational information such as that available at www.nctsn.org.

During psychoeducation for parents, the therapist provides information about the child's trauma experiences and common responses, as described earlier. Important information related to the child's trauma experience may be provided during the psychoeducation component; for example, children who have experienced sexual abuse begin to receive developmentally appropriate information about sexual abuse, including proper names for private parts. Some safety information may be incorporated during the psychoeducation component (eg, doctor's names for private body parts and information about okay and not okay touches for young children who have experienced sexual abuse). However, for children with complex trauma or those at very high risk of experiencing ongoing trauma, the Enhancing Safety component may be provided as the initial TF-CBT component before psychoeducation, as described in detail elsewhere.[11,14,15]

Importantly, the therapist helps the parents begin to identify potential trauma reminders. Trauma reminders are any cue (eg, people, places, situations, sights, smells, memories, internal sensations) that remind the child of an earlier trauma; this initiates a cascade of psychological, physical, and neurobiological responses similar to those the child experienced at the time of the original trauma. When parents understand this process, they can make more sense of children's trauma responses and intervene earlier in the process to support the children's use of TF-CBT skills to interrupt, reverse, or mitigate the process. For example, a child in foster care who had experienced previous domestic violence and physical abuse from his father became angry and aggressive when yelled at by an older foster brother, leading him to hit younger children in the home. For this child, loud or angry voices were trauma reminders of his father (perpetrator), who often screamed before becoming physically abusive. The foster mother yelled at this child when he became aggressive to the younger children, causing him to become even more dysregulated. Psychoeducation about the child's trauma reminders and responses was the first step in changing this pattern.

Parenting Skills

During the parent skills component, parents gain effective strategies for responding to children's behavioral and emotional dysregulation. The therapist typically provides specific instruction, practice, and role plays in parenting skills, which the therapist clinically determines according to the child's presentation and the parents' current knowledge and skills. The therapist always encourages parents to use these skills while remembering that the child's behavioral problems occur in the context of trauma reminders. More detailed information about implementing these skills is available elsewhere.[9,10]

Time in and time out Time out involves placing the child in a quiet place that lacks child-family interaction or other positive stimulation in order to encourage the child to reregulate his or her own emotions and/or behavior. When the larger family context is that the child has frequent positive, nurturing, and enjoyable interactions with parents (time in), the child typically finds time out to be very negative and wants to return to time in as soon as possible. Thus, time out is most effective when the family provides high-quality time in.

Praise, positive attention, selective attention In order to create time in, therapists instruct parents in using praise, positive attention, and selective attention. Elements of effective praise include identifying specific behaviors the parents want the child to continue, labeling these for the child immediately after they occur, and enthusiastically praising these behaviors without taking back the praise with negative statements or qualifications.

Example of ineffective praise Mother (several hours after son takes out garbage when asked): "Thanks for doing your chores. I wish you were always good like that." (Errors: did not label the specific desired behavior; did not provide praise immediately after the behavior occurred; took back the praise with a negative qualifying statement.)

Example of effective praise Mother (immediately after son takes out garbage when asked): "I like how you took out the garbage as soon as I asked you to do it. Thank you so much for doing that!"

Often parents expect, take for granted, and/or ignore children when they are behaving well, and only give attention to negative or problematic behaviors. Because all children crave parental attention, this paradigm tends to reinforce children's negative behaviors; the opposite of what parents intend. In order to reverse this, positive attention requires parents to look for, attend to, and promptly provide positive attention (hugs, high fives, verbal praise, and/or other positive attention) in response to children's positive behaviors. The therapist helps parents to selectively attend to these positive behaviors while paying less attention to minor negative behaviors that, although annoying or irritating, are not dangerous (eg, pestering or intrusive behaviors, rolling eyes) By reinforcing desired behaviors with high levels of attention and not attending to undesired behaviors, parents often see marked improvements in behavioral problems.

For more significant behavioral problems, the therapist helps the parents and child to collaboratively develop an individualized contingency reinforcement program. Such programs address specific behaviors (eg, aggression, sleep problems, sexually inappropriate behaviors), and provide specific contingencies (rewards such as stars; punishments such as loss of access to electronics) if the child does or does not meet the expectations for the number of times the behavior occurs within a given time period (typically 1 day or part of a day). Critical to the success of these programs are to: (1) include the child and parents in developing the program and prizes associated with rewards; (2) chose only 1 behavior to address at a time rather than attempting to resolve multiple behaviors simultaneously; (3) have parents provide praise for any successes and provide contingencies and rewards promptly and consistently.

Relaxation Skills

As noted earlier, traumatized children experience multiple neurobiological changes that tend to maintain trauma responses. Parents may experience their own personal biological hyperarousal responses. Relaxation skills can help children and parents to reregulate these stress systems, both in resting states and in response to trauma reminders. The therapist provides personalized relaxation strategies to the child and encourages them to practice these on a regular basis at home. These strategies may include focused (yoga) breathing, progressive muscle relaxation, and visualization, skills that have been shown to produce physiologic relaxation responses, but therapists may also encourage children to use a variety of other relaxation strategies based on the child's own interests and developmental level. For example, young children often like to relax through blowing bubbles, dance (eg, Hokey Pokey, Chicken Song), and song (Row, Row, Row Your Boat), whereas teens often prefer to relax using their favorite music, physical activities, or crafts, such as crochet or knitting. Other children find reading or prayer relaxing. It is important for children to develop a variety of different relaxation strategies because a particular strategy (eg, exercise) may be effective in some settings (eg, after school or with peers) but not in others (eg, when going to sleep at night).

After the child has identified and practiced several acceptable relaxation strategies, the therapist meets with the parents and teaches them the relaxation skills preferred by the child. The therapist helps the parents to recognize situations in which the child may be experiencing physiologic arousal in response to trauma reminders and encourages the parents to support the child in using the relaxation skills in these situations. Parents often find relaxation skills to help with their personal anxiety or hyperarousal responses and the therapist may encourage parents to use relaxation in this regard as well. As noted earlier, younger children may enjoy demonstrating the newly practiced relaxation skills directly to the parents in a brief joint meeting with the parents at the end of this session.

Affect Modulation Skills

During trauma experiences many children learn to not express, develop distance from, or even deny negative feelings as a self-protective mechanism. During this component the therapist helps children to become comfortable with expressing a variety of different feelings and to develop skills for managing negative affective states. These skills may include strategies such as problem solving, seeking social support, positive distraction techniques (eg, humor, journaling, helping others, perspective taking, reading, taking a walk, playing with a pet), focusing on the present, and a variety of anger management techniques. The therapist encourages the child to develop a tool kit of skills that work in different settings and for different negative feelings.[9] These skills are familiar to most child therapists; however, in contrast with other child treatments, in TF-CBT the therapist encourages the child to implement the affective modulation skills in response to trauma reminders.

After identifying the child's preferred affective modulation strategies, the therapist then educates, practices, and role plays with the parents about how they can support the child in implementing these skills. This process often requires substantial parental tolerance and forbearance.

Helping parents to tolerate children's verbal expressions of negative emotions as a positive step toward improved affective regulation is often challenging for the therapist and parents, especially when the parents' cultural perspective views verbalizations of negative emotions (eg, using cuss words, or saying "I hate you") as disrespectful. Some parents have limited tolerance for their child's demands for parental support, especially when these come at inconvenient times or are viewed as whining or manipulative. The therapist may address this by having the parents keep a chart of the child's negative behaviors and requests for support; such parents often find that negative behaviors occur soon after the child unsuccessfully asks for support, and that if/when the parents begin to respond more consistently to the child's requests for support, the problematic behaviors begin to decrease.

Cognitive Processing Skills

During this component the therapist helps children recognize connections among thoughts, feelings, and behaviors (the cognitive triangle) and replace maladaptive cognitions (inaccurate or unhelpful thoughts) related to everyday events with more accurate or helpful cognitions. At this point in TF-CBT the therapist is not focusing on trauma-related thoughts with the child, because it is more effective to process these during the trauma narrative component. The therapist may use a variety of techniques to assist children with cognitive processing, including progressive logical (Socratic) questioning, responsibility pie, and best friend role play.[9,10]

The therapist meets with the parent to introduce the cognitive triangle and to begin processing the parents' maladaptive cognitions. Initially the therapist identifies parents' maladaptive cognitions related to everyday events and helps the parents use cognitive processing in this regard. Many parents have maladaptive cognitions related to the child's trauma (eg, "I should have protected my child"; "I should have known sooner that this was happening to my child"; "My child is forever damaged because of what happened"). The therapist uses clinical judgment to decide whether to begin processing the parents' trauma-related maladaptive cognitions (ie, before or during the child's trauma narrative). Cognitive processing techniques are described in a free Web-based training site, CPT*Web*, available at www.musc.edu/cpt.

TRAUMA NARRATIVE AND PROCESSING PHASE (4–6 SESSIONS)
Trauma Narrative and Processing

During the trauma narrative and processing phase, the therapist and child engage in an interactive process during which the child describes increasingly difficult details about personal trauma experiences, including thoughts, feelings, and body sensations that occurred during these traumas. Through this process the child speaks about even the most horrific and feared traumatic memories, thus speaking the unspeakable, which enables the child to learn a mastery rather than avoidance response to these memories. Through the process of retelling the story as it is being developed further, the child has multiple opportunities for repeated practice of learning this mastery over traumatic memories; this also enables the child to gain perspective about the trauma experiences and thereby to identify potential errors in beliefs that the child previously assumed to be set in stone (maladaptive cognitions; eg, "I deserved to be abused"). Through the cognitive processing strategies learned previously the therapist helps the child to process trauma-related maladaptive cognitions. The child develops a written summary of the trauma narrative process, usually in the form of a book, poem, or song. However, it is critical to emphasize that this written document is only a small fraction of the trauma narrative, which is an interactive process that occurs between the child and therapist, typically over the course of several sessions. The written narrative often is organized into chapters (eg, "About me"; "How it all began"; "Sexual abuse through the years"; "Domestic violence sucks"; "Death"; "Escape"; "How I've changed"). Children who have experienced complex trauma often develop a life narrative rather than a chapter narrative, organized around a central trauma theme.[11] However, like other TF-CBT trauma narratives, these also describe specific trauma episodes in detail.

As the child meets with the therapist weekly to develop the narrative, the therapist meets in parallel sessions with the parents to share the content of the child's narrative. This sharing serves multiple purposes. Few parents have heard all of the details about the child's trauma experiences, and this process allows the parents to understand the child's trauma experiences more fully. Even when the parent coexperienced the trauma, such as a mother who was the direct victim of domestic violence that the child witnessed, it is common for these perspectives to differ considerably and a primary goal of the TF-CBT process is for nonoffending parents to hear and support the child's personal perspective. Another goal is to help parents to identify and process their personal trauma-related maladaptive cognitions; for example, hearing the child's trauma narrative may cause parents to question why their child did not tell them about the abuse sooner, and this provides an opportunity for the parents to thoroughly process this maladaptive cognition. In addition, hearing the child's trauma narrative in separate sessions with the therapist as the child is developing the narrative provides the parents with adequate time to prepare emotionally and cognitively for the conjoint child-parent sessions, during which the child typically shares the narrative directly with the parents. Through repeated exposure to the child's narrative the parents, like the child, gain new mastery related to hearing about their child's trauma experiences, and thus more ability to model adaptive coping in the child's presence during the conjoint sessions.

INTEGRATION AND CONSOLIDATION PHASE (4–6 SESSIONS)
In Vivo Mastery

In vivo mastery is the only optional TF-CBT component. Some children develop ongoing fears and avoidance of situations that are inherently innocuous. When this avoidance significantly interferes with children's adaptive functioning, it becomes an important issue to address in treatment; TF-CBT therapists use clinical judgment to determine which children require this component. For example, a child who was sexually abused in her bedroom by a perpetrator who is no longer in the home was still afraid to sleep in her own bed, and eventually afraid to sleep at night at all, and was disrupting other family members' sleep. Another child who witnessed his sibling's sudden death at home avoided attending school for fear that his mother or another younger sibling would also die when he was not home. In vivo mastery would be appropriate for these children. In distinction to the trauma narrative, which involves imaginal exposure to children's trauma experiences, in vivo (in real life) mastery involves exposure to the innocuous situation (eg, sleeping in one's own bed; returning to school) that the child fears and avoids. Through gradually facing the feared situation and learning that the feared outcome does not happen, the child learns mastery rather than avoidance.

In order to implement in vivo mastery, the therapist, child, and parents develop a fear hierarchy (sometimes referred to as a fear ladder), ascending from the least feared (1) to most feared (10) scenarios, with 10 being the desired end point (eg, the child sleeping in her own bed or attending full days of school). In vivo mastery involves gradually building up to or mastering the end point through mastering a series of smaller steps. Because in vivo mastery typically takes several weeks to complete and also because the child's adaptive functioning is significantly affected, the therapist usually begins in vivo mastery during the TF-CBT stabilization skills phase. Because relaxation and other TF-CBT stabilization skills are needed to help the child (and often the parent) to tolerate the intermediate steps in the fear hierarchy, the therapist often provides psychoeducation, parenting skills, and relaxation skills before initiating the in vivo mastery plan.

The parents are critical to the success of in vivo mastery. Children are often reluctant to surrender the fears that they believe are keeping bad things from happening and parents provide confidence and reassurance that helps the child to get through the difficult early stages of the mastery process. Parents and (if applicable) school personnel must understand why in vivo mastery is important to the child's improved adaptive functioning and must join in with the plan for it to be successful. The therapist must address the parents' concerns or fears about the child gaining mastery over the feared situation, as well as any potential secondary gain that parents may derive from the child continuing the avoidant behavior. The therapist also encourages the parents to use ongoing praise, patience, and persistence in encouraging the child to use relaxation and other TF-CBT skills during the in vivo mastery plan. These skills increasingly reap rewards for the child and parents as the child gains increasing pride in mastering previously feared situations. If the parents do not perform the in vivo plan consistently, the child's fear and avoidance often get even worse, because of the power of intermittent reinforcement. The therapist should not embark on an in vivo plan unless the parents are fully invested in seeing the plan through to completion.

Conjoint Child-Parent Sessions

The therapist provides several conjoint child-parent sessions during the integration and consolidation phase. These sessions provide opportunities for modeling and optimizing direct communication among family members about the child's traumatic experiences and other important topics before treatment closure. During conjoint sessions the therapist typically meets briefly with the parents alone (5–10 minutes) and the child alone (5–10 minutes) to prepare each for the rest of the session (conjoint child-parent session, 40–50 minutes).

The first conjoint session is usually devoted to the child sharing the trauma narrative. If this occurs, the parents have already heard and cognitively processed the child's narrative during their individual parent sessions with the therapist (described earlier). In addition to the child sharing the narrative, the child and parents may ask each other several questions that they prepared during their respective preparation time. For example, one child asked his parents "How were you feeling when I disclosed the sexual abuse"; a parent asked her son, "Did you ever blame me for your sister's death?" These questions often facilitate open discussion of deeper feelings and cognitions related to the child's trauma experiences and many families report that these sessions were the most valuable part of their TF-CBT treatment.

Subsequent conjoint child-parent sessions may address healthy sexuality, bullying prevention, substance use refusal skills, making good peer or dating decisions, enhancing family communication, enhancing safety, or other topics according to the therapist's clinical judgment. For children who have experienced sexual abuse it is particularly important for therapists to address healthy sexuality, and parents often prefer to be included in this process. Whatever the topic the therapist selects, it is helpful to make the process fun and interactive rather than didactic. For example, most children enjoy competing with their parents in quiz or other games in which they can display their increasing knowledge and understanding about trauma and its impact. During the conjoint sessions the therapist may reintroduce What Do You Know or other therapeutic games used earlier in TF-CBT to use in this regard.

Enhancing Safety

Because traumatic experiences involve the loss of safety and betrayal of trust, it is important for children and parents to acknowledge this openly during treatment and to develop practical strategies for enhancing children's physical safety as well as emotional and interactive means for enhancing the child's internal sense of security and trust. In cases in which there is ongoing risk of trauma exposure, the safety component is addressed at the beginning and often throughout TF-CBT.[11,14,15] Whether or not there is risk of repeated trauma exposure, it is usually helpful to develop a systematic family safety plan that applies to all family members, which might include no violence, no substance abuse, no secrets (ie, everyone tells and no one keeps secrets related to breaking the family safety rules), and other mutually agreed-on rules that help all family members to feel safe within the home. Communicating these to all family members and practicing their implementation at home enhances the child's belief that everyone in the family will adhere to the safety plan.

EVALUATION OF OUTCOME

TF-CBT has been evaluated in 15 randomized controlled trials in which it was compared with other active treatments/usual community care (in clinical settings) or wait-list control conditions (in refugee or war conditions). Among the currently evidence-based child trauma treatments, TF-CBT alone has been evaluated across the child and adolescent developmental spectrum (3–18 years), for multiple index trauma types (eg, sexual abuse, commercial sexual exploitation, domestic violence, disaster, war, traumatic grief, multiple and complex trauma), in different settings (eg, clinic, foster care, community domestic violence center, refugee nongovernmental organization, human immunodeficiency virus treatment centers), and in multiple countries and cultures (eg, United States, Africa, Europe, Australia) and with both mental health and non–mental health providers. In all of these studies TF-CBT has been found to be superior to the comparison conditions for improving PTSD symptoms/diagnosis, as well as other related mental health difficulties, such as depressive, anxiety, behavioral, cognitive, relationship, and other problems.

In many of these studies the impact of including parents in treatment has been examined. One study compared TF-CBT provided to child only, parent only, or child plus parent, with usual community treatment.[16] The TF-CBT conditions that included the parent led to significantly greater improvement in positive parenting practices as well as in the child's behavioral problems and child-reported depressive problems. A study of preschoolers who had experienced sexual abuse documented that TF-CBT led to greater improvement in child outcomes as well as in parental support and parental emotional distress than nondirective supportive therapy. Improvement in parental support significantly mediated improvement in children's PTSD symptoms after treatment and improvement in parental support and emotional distress significantly mediated improvement in children's behavioral problems at 6-month and 12-month follow-ups.[17,18] A study of children aged 8 to 14 years who experienced sexual abuse showed that TF-CBT led to significantly greater improvement in parental support and this improvement significantly mediated improvement in children's depressive and anxiety symptoms.[19] Recent research has shown that including foster parents in TF-CBT enhanced the foster parent's engagement in treatment and the family's retention in treatment.[20,21] A recent community treatment study in Norway comparing TF-CBT with usual care found that, in addition to children in the TF-CBT group experiencing significantly greater improvement in PTSD, general mental health symptoms, and functional impairment,[22] parents in the TF-CBT condition experienced significantly greater improvement in their personal depressive symptoms and this mediated significantly greater improvement in children's depressive symptoms in the TF-CBT condition only.[23]

SUMMARY

TF-CBT is a family-based treatment of traumatized children with strong empirical support for improving PTSD, depressive, anxiety, behavioral, cognitive, relationship, and other problems. Parents or caregivers participate in all components of TF-CBT during initial parallel individual parent sessions and later conjoint parent-child sessions. Several studies document that parental inclusion significantly contributes to positive child outcomes.

REFERENCES

1. Copeland W, Keeler G, Angold A, et al. Traumatic events and post-traumatic stress in childhood. Arch Gen Psychiatry 2007;64:577–84.
2. Felitti VJ, Anda RF, Nordenberg D, et al. Relationship of childhood abuse and household dysfunction to many of the leading causes of death in adults. The Adverse Childhood Experiences (ACE) Study. Am J Prev Med 1998;14(4): 245–58.
3. Kilpatrick D, Ruggiero KJ, Acierno R, et al. Violence and risk of PTSD, major depression, substance abuse/dependence and comorbidity: results for the National Survey of Adolescents. J Consult Clin Psychol 2003;71:692–700.
4. Pine DC, Cohen JA. Trauma in children: risk and treatment of psychiatric sequelae. Biol Psychiatry 2002;51:519–31.
5. Kisiel C, Conradi L, Gehernbach T, et al. Assessing the effects of trauma in children and adolescents in practice settings. Child Adolesc Psychiatr Clin N Am 2014;23:223–42.
6. Mannarino AP, Cohen JA. Treating sexually abused children and their families: identifying and avoiding professional role conflicts. Trauma Violence Abuse 2001;2:331–42.
7. Steinberg AM, Brymer MJ, Decker K, et al. The University of California at Los Angeles Posttraumatic Stress Disorder Reaction Index. Curr Psychiatry Rep 2004;6: 96–100.
8. Foa EB, Treadwell K, Johnson K, et al. The child PTSD symptom scale: a preliminary examination of its psychometric properties. J Clin Child Psychol 2001;30: 376–84.
9. Cohen JA, Mannarino AP, Deblinger E. Treating trauma and traumatic grief in children and adolescents. New York: Guilford Press; 2006.
10. Cohen JA, Mannarino AP, Deblinger E, editors. Trauma-focused CBT for children and adolescents: treatment applications. New York: Guilford Press; 2012.

11. Cohen JA, Mannarino AP, Kleithermes M, et al. Trauma-focused cognitive behavioral therapy for youth with complex trauma. Child Abuse Negl 2012;36:528–41.
12. Craske MG, Kircanshi K, Zelikowski M, et al. Optimizing inhibitory learning during exposure therapy. Behav Res Ther 2008;46:5–27.
13. CARES Institute. What do you know? Stratford (NJ): Rowan University; 2006.
14. Cohen JA, Mannarino AP, Murray LK. Trauma-focused CBT for youth who experience ongoing traumas. Child Abuse Negl 2011;35:637–46.
15. Murray LK, Cohen JA, Mannarino AP. Trauma-focused CBT for youth who experience continuous traumatic stress. Peace Confl 2013;19:180–95.
16. Deblinger E, Lippmann J, Steer RA. Sexually abused children suffering posttraumatic stress symptoms: initial treatment outcome findings. Child Maltreat 1996;1: 310–21.
17. Cohen JA, Mannarino AP. A treatment outcome study for sexually abused preschool children: initial findings. J Am Acad Child Adolesc Psychiatry 1996;35: 42–50.
18. Cohen JA, Mannarino AP. Factors that mediate treatment outcome of sexually abused preschoolers: six and twelve month follow-ups. J Am Acad Child Adolesc Psychiatry 1998;37:44–51.
19. Cohen JA, Mannarino AP. Predictors of treatment outcome in sexually abused children. Child Abuse Negl 2000;24:983–94.
20. Dorsey S, Pullmann MD, Berliner L, et al. Engaging foster parents in treatment: a randomized trial of supplementing trauma-focused cognitive behavioral therapy with evidence-based engagement strategies. Child Abuse Negl 2014;38: 1508–20.
21. Dorsey S, Conover K, Cox JR. Improving foster parent engagement: using qualitative methods to guide tailoring of evidence-based engagement strategies. J Clin Child Adolesc Psychol, in press.
22. Jensen TK, Holt T, Ormhaug SM, et al. A randomized effectiveness study comparing trauma-focused cognitive behavioral therapy with therapy as usual for youth. J Clin Child Adolesc Psychol 2013;43:356–69.
23. Holt T, Jensen TK, Wentzel-Larsen T. The change and the mediating role of parental emotional reactions and depression in the treatment of traumatized youth: results from a randomized controlled study. Child Adolesc Psychiatry Ment Health 2014;8:11.

Family System Interventions for Families of Children with Autism Spectrum Disorder

Eric Goepfert, MD[a],*, Christina Mulé, PhD[a], Erik von Hahn, MD[a], Zachary Visco, BA[a], Matthew Siegel, MD[b]

KEYWORDS

- Family therapy • Autism spectrum disorder • Family system

KEY POINTS

- Few empirical family therapy studies have been conducted with children diagnosed with autism spectrum disorder (ASD) and their families.
- Despite the lack of a rigorous evidence base, families with ASD can benefit from family therapy or from care informed by family systems theory.
- Although family therapy cannot alter ASD or eliminate its presence, it may improve relationships and the strength of the system living with ASD.
- Family therapy can repair and strengthen relationships, and can help family members to better collaborate with one another and providers in supporting the child, thus positively affecting child outcomes.
- Family therapy can foster a perspective of hope and empowerment that maximizes the child's success.

Since the diagnosis of autism spectrum disorder (ASD) was first described,[1] a considerable body of research has taught clinicians much about the neurobiology, behavioral features, and appropriate treatments for children with ASD. In spite of this, families continue to struggle when their children are diagnosed with ASD, and many children with ASD do not reach their full potential. Although it is appropriate and important for clinicians to understand the science of ASD and its treatments, the focus of this article is to help the reader apply principles of family systems thinking in those cases in which a family and child with ASD are not functioning well, in spite of appropriate treatments that the child may be receiving.

Disclosure: The authors have nothing to disclose.
[a] Pediatrics and Child and Adolescent Psychiatry, Tufts Medical Center, 800 Washington Street, Boston, MA 02111, USA; [b] Maine Medical Center Research Institute, 81 Research Drive, Scarborough, ME 04074, USA
* Corresponding author. 800 Washington Street, #345, Boston, MA 02111.
E-mail address: egoepfert@tuftsmedicalcenter.org

Child Adolesc Psychiatric Clin N Am 24 (2015) 571–583
http://dx.doi.org/10.1016/j.chc.2015.02.009
1056-4993/15/$ – see front matter © 2015 Elsevier Inc. All rights reserved.

Abbreviations	
ASD	Autism spectrum disorder
DSM-5	Diagnostic and Statistical Manual for Mental Health Disorders, 5th Edition
MFT	Medical family therapy
MST	Multisystemic therapy

The traditional medical model emphasizes a linear model of thinking, outlining symptoms, illnesses, and diagnoses defined by scientific inquiry. Specialists make the diagnosis and recommend treatment. Multiple providers provide expert assessments and subsequent plans to the families, but the families may have little input. This medical model works well for many biological conditions, but has limitations for behavioral health conditions.

Providers practicing family therapy have moved away from this linear, hierarchical medical model. Instead, family systems–oriented therapists seek to help families construct their own truths about themselves within their contexts; a concept called social constructionism.[2] The process of family therapy is nonlinear, meaning that feedback between families and providers (shared decision making) determines what the treatment should be. Client empowerment and other patient-centered outcomes (ie, quality of life), in addition to symptom reduction, signify treatment success.

Although the child's diagnosis of ASD cannot be changed, the family's responses to the diagnosis and challenges of ASD are malleable. Families describe their experiences (their truths) in narratives. All providers cocreate narratives with their clients at every encounter. Narrative therapists, a distinct school of family therapy, aim to change narratives themselves, through exploring how stories are prioritized, what aspects are prioritized, what words are used, and the meanings therein. Although this article discuses narrative therapy in more detail, it is introduced here in order to prime the reader's frame of mind to think about families' narratives describing their lives with a child with ASD. In addition, specific schools of family therapy are not reviewed exhaustively.

CLINICAL CONSIDERATIONS
Diagnostic Criteria and Clinical Description

ASD is a lifelong neurodevelopmental disorder characterized in the *Diagnostic and Statistical Manual for Mental Health Disorders, 5th Edition* (DSM-5) by deficits that impair everyday functioning in 2 core domains: (1) significant impairments in social communication and interaction across contexts; and (2) restricted, repetitive patterns of behaviors, interests, and/or activities.[3] For providers who are unfamiliar with this population, it is difficult to imagine or picture children with ASD merely by reading the description provided in the DSM-5. Children with ASD present with a spectrum of impairments and can look different from one another. Deficits in social communication range from a child who is nonverbal to one who is highly verbal with subtle impairments in social pragmatics. Repetitive behaviors and interests extend from all-consuming stimulatory behaviors to mild preoccupations with certain topics or activities.

Comorbidity

In addition to the core features, comorbid psychiatric conditions are common among individuals with ASD.[4] These conditions include attention deficit hyperactivity disorder, disruptive behavior disorders, anxiety disorders, and depression.[5] Some of these comorbid conditions only become evident as the child with ASD ages into adolescence, but can obscure an accurate diagnosis at any age.[6] Coupled with comorbid conditions, ASD can result in significant treatment challenges,[7] psychiatric hospitalizations, polypharmacy,[8] and risk of poor health outcomes. The deficits of ASD persist into adulthood, and make it difficult for individuals with ASD at the more severe end of the spectrum to live independently.[9] As a consequence, they often experience reduced quality of life compared with their neurotypical peers.[10]

Individual Interventions

The variability and comorbidity of ASD complicate choosing interventions. Many child-centered, individual interventions have been developed and are offered to improve skills and reduce the symptoms associated with ASD.[11] Common treatments include applied behavioral analysis[12]; numerous developmental approaches (eg, the Early Start Denver Model; and developmental, individual-difference, relationships-based therapy, known as floor time)[13,14]; as well as therapies with other specific goals, such as social skills training,[15] occupational therapy/sensory integration therapy,[16] and speech and language therapy.[17] Pharmacologic treatments are also used in children with ASD to target the various comorbid conditions. Children with ASD commonly receive many interventions simultaneously, and health care service use is high.[18] Treatments and services are often uncoordinated, because they are delivered by distinct agencies (health system, educational system, state agencies). These services consume significant internal and external resources (eg, emotional and financial) from both the child and family.[19]

IMPACT ON THE FAMILY: A NARRATIVE

A diagnosis of ASD brings myriad challenges to both the individual children and their families. The family's narrative of having a child with ASD can play a supportive or a debilitating role in the outcome for the child and family.

Impact of Diagnosis

A family's narrative begins before the child's birth, as parents create expectations and assumptions about who their child will be. These expectations and assumptions come into question when the child is noted to be developing differently. This difficult process may be made worse by a nonresponsive care system (eg, when the family is told by their child's doctor to wait and see; when the family does not have access to specialist care for a formal diagnosis; or when the family may defer specialist evaluation because of their own uncertainty, denial, or fear). Once a formal diagnosis is made and information is garnered, the family may be better able to evaluate the assumptions and expectations they had about their child. The conflict between the imagined and the real often creates a crisis.

For some families the journey after the diagnosis is more linear and expectable. Accepting the diagnosis facilitates a continued positive attachment with the child and promotes successful working relationships with providers. Other families may struggle. The seemingly vague diagnostic criteria can make it difficult to accept the diagnosis, to make informed treatment choices, and to incorporate those treatments into day-to-day life. Interventions and services may reinforce the (often mistaken) belief that the parents do not know how to parent their own child. Each unreached developmental milestone may remind the family of the loss of the child they envisioned, resulting in a prolonged or repeated grief reaction.

Some families have additional factors complicating their experience and the narrative they create about their child. These factors can include stressors such as poverty, other children with special needs, lack of community supports, or cultural shame. The family's response to diagnosis often influences how they manage future disappointments or problems. Healing takes time and resourcefulness, and past traumas may impede healing. Where a family is in the process of healing affects the kind of help they want or need (eg, concrete tasks and plans, or attention to their emotions).

Raising a Child with Autism Spectrum Disorder

The deficit-focused diagnostic criteria of ASD, and the problem-oriented focus of most treatments for ASD, can obscure the fact that children with ASD are still children. The child's parents may not attend to daily routines (ie, having fun together, sleeping and eating routines, physical activity, predictable schedules, rules, friendships, home-work), exacerbating the child's performance difficulties and reducing the family's quality of life. Although children with ASD need more dense teaching to learn routines and to participate in the activities of a family, they need those routines as much as any other child.

Even when the family can attend to the routine expectations of parenthood, parenting a child with ASD imposes a considerable burden. The many treatments involved are time consuming: on average, the equivalent of a full-time position.[20] Thus, parents of a child with ASD often have less time for activities that previously filled their lives (eg, paid employment, recreation, self-care).[21] Families can undergo substantial loss of annual household income,[22] have difficulty finding accommodating employment,[23] and have higher rates of parenting stress and mental health problems.[24,25]

Building a Team

The stressors described earlier can be mitigated when the family is able to build a team of helping providers. However, access to care varies by state and between school districts, insurance providers, and different socioeconomic and racial groups. Even after a team of providers is established, many families find it difficult to work with multiple providers working for disparate organizations, each with its own mandates, policies, and constraints that interfere with coordination of care. Recommendations between providers working in different settings may differ or even contradict one another. Providers often have a problem-oriented focus that may or may not be patient or family centered. Further, many families experience staff turnover, and have difficulty accessing care. When families express their frustration, they may be regarded as difficult.

Relationship Strain and Social Isolation

Unsurprisingly, relationships suffer. Parents of children with ASD commonly experience marital strain,[26] report lower marital happiness,[27] and are nearly twice as likely to divorce as parents without a child with ASD.[28] Relationship strain can occur with siblings, who may vie for parental attention, adopt a caregiver role, or hide their own concerns and needs for fear of burdening their parents.[29]

In addition to relationship strain within the nuclear family, parents often find themselves isolated from their extended social support network (ie, their extended family and friends).[30] Parents of children with ASD may avoid social gatherings because of concerns regarding their child's behavior. Parents may feel shame or blame themselves for difficulties that their child has. Social isolation also occurs because of a lack of understanding and awareness in the community and the limited number of places that might be friendly toward a child with ASD. This self-imposed sequestration results in parents routinely thinking that they are unsupported or isolated in their quest to parent a child with ASD. Despite this, families may form very bolstering relationships with providers of care for their child, and these can become a new support network.

FAMILY APPROACHES TO MANAGEMENT

As stated previously, family therapy does not cure ASD. It seeks to help families by examining relationships and the broader context of their lives. Children with ASD are decentralized as the problem, and the problem is reframed instead as a pattern of interactions between people (in systems terms). For such a reframe to be effective, it must be unanimously true to all involved family members, which requires an alliance between the provider and each member, and it requires that the provider shows understanding of some aspect of each person's experience; this is called multipartiality, and it serves to prioritize no 1 individual's perspective. Multipartial, nonpejorative, systemic reframes often allow issues to be more openly discussed (see case 1 for an illustrative example). Multiple members of a family are involved in the problem and therefore share responsibility for changing it.

CASE 1. MULTIPARTIAL STANCE AND REDEFINITION OF THE PROBLEM IN SYSTEMS TERMS

Background

Mr and Mrs Matthews had both emigrated from South Africa to the United States, where they married and had 2 children. Their son, Paul, has high-functioning ASD. They have been in treatment with a developmental pediatrician, and Mrs Matthews has been in individual therapy, but Mr Matthews has never been interested in behavioral health interventions. Paul is an affable boy who has always made progress in school. However, he has difficulty with daily routines at home, and his parents disagree about what approach is best. Their pediatrician recommended more dense structure in expectations and strategies to decrease reliance on tangible rewards, but the family had not implemented these suggestions.

Family Systems Formulation

At the beginning of the first session, while her husband is parking the car, Mrs Matthews refers to her husband as violent. This word raises our team's anxiety, and we defer discussion until he joins us. Intending to be multipartial, rather than siding with 1 parent, we explore the reasons behind her accusation of violence. Mr Matthews' father had left his family when he was a child. Mr Matthews became a caretaker in the home, prizing tidiness, thriving on structure, and treasuring the calm sense of things being okay. He becomes angry when things are not structured or tidy enough, and when he feels ineffective. Mrs Matthews' mother was severely depressed and often neglected her daughter's needs. Mrs Matthews thus sought validation outside the home. Her spontaneity still keeps her busy, fulfilled, and engaged with the outside world.

We redefine the issues in systems terms. He believes structure is nurturing and necessary, and indeed a grade-school child with ASD needs more structure. However, she avoids causing distress to her children for fear that she was repeating her own painful childhood. When she has a concern in more of an emotional realm, he does not acknowledge the concern unless it disrupts the organization of their home. However, his nonresponse triggers his wife's history of neglect, causing her more distress. She thus increases the volume of her concerns, in order to be heard.

Discussion

Our multipartial and systemic redefinition decreases blame and both parents are engaged in the therapy. We foster mutual understanding so that their disparate approaches are appreciated in their context, rather than viewed as opposition or criticism, which allows them to work more collaboratively and stop cycles of escalating intensity. They are able to start designing uniform parenting strategies and appreciating each other's approach.

Family therapy ameliorates symptoms and improves experiences by helping families to understand how they interact with one another and how they view their children's ASD. By exploring small interactions, family therapy helps to break impossible, big problems down into manageable ones. It identifies small positive gains and amplifies them. It should venture to change the child's environment in order to better accommodate his or her idiosyncrasies, while not doing harm to functional family relationships and structure. The clinician does not act in an authoritarian manner and does not unilaterally prescribe interventions. Rather, the clinician follows the family's agenda, coconstructing each step of therapy, especially when the family moves to shift entrenched relational patterns.

FOUNDATIONAL THEORIES OF FAMILY THERAPY IN THE CONTEXT OF AUTISM SPECTRUM DISORDER

There is no empirically validated family therapy treatment of problems associated with ASD, but many therapists have done family therapy with families that have a child with ASD. Most modern therapists integrate the historically different schools of family therapy. The following presents key concepts from individual schools of family therapy and the application thereof in the context of ASD.

Strategic Therapy

Strategic family therapy originated with the study of communication and feedback loops.[31] Certain responses to problems maintain the status quo of the family and maintain the problem. Expectations about change are managed so that progress is possible and incremental. Based on observations of patterns, strategic therapists design intentionally jarring strategic interventions that serve to create different interactions that change patterns and, it is hoped, decrease problematic interactions. However, change causes stress, and people often revert back to more comfortable and familiar, but problematic, interactions.

Parents often think that they are helpless to change behavior viewed as part of ASD. Strategic approaches may help parents challenge this notion. For example, a strategic therapist might prescribe the symptom, instructing the family to enact the child's usual behavior and their typical responses, and then to evaluate the fidelity of their enactment. Through this, they may learn that behaviors can be changed, planned responses are less impassioned, and predictable problems are less disruptive. In another example, parents may disagree about whether rigid structure or offering choices is the best approach to avert difficult behavior. By asking them to try each approach, every other day, while one parent supports the other without criticism, the therapist may help the parents clarify whether one approach is better. In addition, prescribing rituals (not unique to strategic therapy) can help parents make sense of their situation. Examples of this are a symbolic letting go of the idealized, typical child, or an informational party for friends or family to build a resisting-despair, building-hope team.[32] In all of these examples, insight and internal change may follow, but are not necessary in order to shift external interactions or behaviors (see case 2 for an illustrative example).

CASE 2. CASE EXAMPLE OF A STRATEGIC INTERVENTION FOR DISPARATE PARENTING STYLES

Background

Mr Walcott and Mr Castillo come to clinic with their 9-year-old son, Pedro, who has ASD and mild intellectual disability. He throws severe tantrums that can become aggressive. Pedro is getting bigger and has bitten both parents and his older sister, Alice. Mr Castillo, an engineer, thinks that he has better success with his parenting approach of structure and not bending rules in response to Pedro's behavior. Mr Walcott has resigned from his job as an office manager to care for their children, and he thinks that giving choices is nurturing and helps redirect a tantrum behavior.

Mr Castillo thinks that Pedro may eventually need to be put into a residential setting. Mr Walcott firmly opposes this option. However, both of them are committed to not abandoning the other in what they agree is a 2-person job. Pedro's sister, Alice, has also developed increasing somatic symptoms, which seemed to be caused by her fathers' distress and distraction about Pedro. The fathers want behavior solutions, but they have seen several behaviorists who collected data but whose recommendations were not helpful. They acknowledge the growing animosity between them calmly: "We know we aren't getting along—that's not what we're here to talk about. Give us ideas for Pedro."

Family Systems Formulation

In a usual interaction around Pedro's difficulties, one father criticizes the other. Mutual criticism constrains their thinking, and the growing distance between them engenders more criticism. The more one parent is rigid, the more the other is lenient. Prior therapists' provision of behavioral interventions has neglected the parents' partnership and their different ideas about parenting, which affects the effectiveness of interventions.

Discussion

Although there are many possible avenues of intervention, in this case we elect to focus on an obstacle to their success: their disparate approach prevents learning by the child and limits mutual support between them. To align with their request for directive strategies, we recommend that they take charge of Pedro on alternate days, each supporting his partner without criticism.

They tried the intervention. Neither approach was better, but their relationship improved. Each felt truly supported by the other, and this support engendered flexibility and creativity. Together, they have developed several new, effective solutions, and the child's tantrums have improved.

See **Fig. 1** for further discussion of this case.

Intergenerational/Bowenian Therapy

Bowen[33] developed intergenerational theory, in which a person's emotional coping style is learned in the family of origin. A multigenerational history elucidates possible reasons why people are stuck, because of rules of interaction transmitted implicitly within the family. Differentiation describes the degree to which people achieve their own identity separate from their families, including independence in life, emotions, ideas, and relationships. If differentiation is not allowed or fostered, as a response to fusion, people may remain too close or very distant from their families. A child with ASD has a biologically challenged capacity for development, and practitioners should be wary of attributing insufficient differentiation to family functioning; particularly because psychiatry already has an unfortunate history of blaming families (eg, refrigerator-mother theory as the basis of ASD). However, when a child's ability is greater than that perceived by caregivers, differentiation may be inadequately fostered. A bowenian therapist clarifies roles of family members with respect to the child's disability, considering the family's history of fusion versus differentiation.

Structural Therapy

Structural family theory proposes that symptoms are expressions of structural problems within the family.[34] In order to learn about family structure, structural family

Organizing Vision
Where would you like to be headed in your life?

We want our family to have fun together and support each other
We want our children to do the best they can
We would like to feel calmer when things get difficult
We want effective strategies to manage Pedro's behavior

Obstacles	Supports
What gets in the way?	What helps you get there?
Alice's health problems Our relationship is not good We have different approaches Sometimes it's hard to enjoy time with Pedro	We are committed to our family We believe there is a solution We have people who can help us if we ask them

Plan
What needs to happen next?

To see whether one of the strategies works better, try using each other's strategies every other day. Only support the other without criticism. Think about how it feels to be supported by your partner.

(Although this plan is directive in nature, the process through which we decided upon it was collaborative. As discussed earlier, we followed the parent's wish for specific strategies. However, we thought that the parental tension was a significant obstacle to the couple having their own success, but they were not interested in discussing their relationship. The strategic intervention therefore was intended to decrease their mutual criticism and help them work as a team. Thus, when they experienced successes, the credit was theirs.)

Fig. 1. Collaborative helping map, applied to case 2. (*Adapted from* Madsen WC. Collaborative therapy with multi-stressed families. 2nd edition. New York: The Guildford Press; 2007.)

therapists may prescribe and observe tasks, called enactments, given to the family in session. For example, a therapist may ask a family to plan a trip that everyone will enjoy. They then observe who talks to whom and how they do so, who makes decisions, how they manage conflict, and what alliances exist. The response to the task can help show how the family interacts with the outside world (see case 3 for an illustrative example). For example, a child's increasing symptoms (eg, anxiety or somatization) may decrease parental conflict or distance, or the child may be take charge (eg, tantrum) when parents disagree or set limits ineffectively. Shifting this dysfunctional structure may improve symptoms.

CASE 3. CASE EXAMPLE OF A STRUCTURAL FAMILY THERAPY FORMULATION

Background

The Costas bring Anna, their daughter with ASD and borderline cognitive functioning, to understand why a variety of medications have not been helpful. Anna has increased oppositionality and tantrums at home, most often when her parents are busy doing other things, including helping her sister, 11-year-old Daniella, with her homework. A prior behaviorist correctly identified that the more the parents attended to her tantrums, the more often they occurred. The behaviorist recommended planned ignoring as a new response. However, the Costas have not had much success implementing this strategy.

Family Systems Formulation

Anna's developmental stage allows a growing awareness of her differences from her peers. She has difficulty making friends, and school is more and more challenging. We learn also that her parents both work as advocates for the mentally ill. In the context of these factors, Anna effectively controls her home environment through her tantrums and oppositionality. Given her disability and their professional work, Anna's parents experience planned ignoring as being neglectful. We invite Daniella to join us for the intake, in which an enactment (asking each member to suggest a vacation that everyone will enjoy) shows us that Daniella tends to subjugate her own needs to look after Anna and avoid creating strain between her parents.

Discussion

Through an enactment, we learn patterns of interaction and roles within the family. We challenge the assumption that the Costas are being neglectful, and we redefine limits and planned ignoring as nurturing for Anna, who likely feels overwhelmed with the power she has. The Costas are then able to try these evidence-based interventions. Anna's tantrums decrease, and her parents think that they are more in control of their family. They intentionally attend to Daniella's needs, and the calmer environment allows Daniella to share her difficulties with her parents. The parents have reestablished their authority and their responsibility for caring for their children.

Structural theories are highly applicable to ASD. The most common potentially problematic structure of families of children with ASD occurs when 1 parent orchestrates most of the child's care and activities. This intensive involvement may be necessary, but it becomes difficult for the other parent to know how to be helpful, and may result in increased distance and anguish in the couple. Each partner may soothe their anguish by immersing themselves more deeply in their respective work, stabilizing the distance between the couple and the overinvolvement of 1 parent with the child. Acknowledging this pattern and building a parenting partnership with more equitable involvement in the care of the child improves the mutual support, intimacy, stamina, and flexibility of the couple. This improvement engenders the creativity that is necessary in parenting a child with special needs.

Psychodynamic Therapy

A psychodynamic family therapist helps family members develop insight into the individual's internal psyches. A person's psyche is influenced by prior generations' experiences, including trauma and illness; by attachment styles from one generation to the next; and by other individual subconscious factors that may not have origins in the family's history. With regard to ASD, the child's biology impedes development of reciprocal interactions, which can affect development of attachment. Psychodynamic therapists facilitate attachment by helping parents improve connections to their children, appreciating children's social cognitive abilities, and also considering the parents' own histories of attachment.

Narrative Therapy

Families have been taught to bring problem-focused accounts to providers' offices. Less attention is paid to the concurrent accounts of strengths and abilities. However, these less available accounts may be the means through which therapeutic improvements happen. Narrative therapists craft conversations to help families reconnect with aspects of their experience that show their abilities to manage problems successfully.[35] There are few studied applications of narrative therapy in the context of

ASD,[36] but many narrative concepts are relevant. Narrative therapists may externalize the problem: the problem is named and separated from the individual and family, in order to assess how the problem affects them and how they affect the problem. A therapist may externalize the ASD, a comorbid behavioral problem, society's perception of ASD, or even the family's grief in response to the ASD. Externalization separates blame from responsibility (ie, behaviors are not simply caused by bad children or ineffective parents).[37]

Central to narrative therapy interventions are reflections offered by providers to families.[38] These reflections, either verbal or written, do not formulate reasons for problems, and they do not advise. Rather, they attend to and augment the alternative stories that show the coping and resourcefulness of the family's response to ASD. The family's response to the clinicians' reflections minimizes hierarchy and optimizes collaboration (see case 4 for an illustrative example).

CASE 4. CASE EXAMPLE OF USING REFLECTION TO CHANGE A NARRATIVE

Background

The Conways have 5 adopted children, 3 of whom have ASD. They have an excellent support network, and they are strong advocates for ASD in their community. They present to clinic when their 15-year-old son, Mark, who they describe as their highest functioning child, shows new behaviors. Although they are experts at managing issues for their children, his new behaviors are more severe, disruptive, and difficult than before, and they are not sure what to do.

Family Systems Formulation

His behaviors challenge these expert parents' narrative of themselves as effective and creative, which leaves them feeling hopeless. We invite them to respond to the following question: are they indeed hopeless, or do they need to find new ways to deal with new difficulties? We also reflect to them what we see and invite them to respond. They have not realized that they felt hopeless. At the next meeting, they have tweaked routines around bedtime and community outings to help their son manage himself, and the disruptive episodes have decreased significantly.

Discussion

Naming hopelessness moved them away from shame and fear and reconnected them to their expertise, with which they crafted new solutions. Had we simply given ideas for behavior management, we may have undermined their authority and expertise with their son. The obstacle to their vision, to feel effective at managing their children's difficulties, was in the meaning they attributed to the new symptoms. Our meetings helped by shifting this narrative.

Other schools of family therapy deserving of mention

Multisystemic therapy (MST; discussed by Zajac and colleagues elsewhere in this issue), which was developed and validated rigorously for conduct problems, is an intensive treatment that contends that behaviors are determined by multiple overlapping contexts (family, community, school), and that behaviors improve through changes in each. Dysfunctional contexts do not cause ASD. However, behaviors may persist and skills may not generalize if there is not a uniform approach in the child's multiple environments. Wagner and colleagues[19] (2012) adapted MST for behavior problems in the context of ASD.

Medical family therapy (MFT) integrates family therapy into medical care, and a substantial body of research shows its benefits. MFT therapists use a biopsychosocial approach to integrate linear medicine with nonlinear systems theory. This approach elicits an illness story, removes blame and respects defenses, follows the family's agency, and attends to developmental issues.[39] However, it does not aim to change the narrative, as does narrative therapy.

THERAPY IN PRACTICE

This article provides a basic foundation for conducting family therapy in the context of ASD. However, therapy seldom follows a map, and it can be difficult to know where to start. Madsen[40] (2007) provides a helpful framework for organizing collaborative work. He recommends the use of collaborative helping maps, whereby families define their vision for their near future (what they would like for themselves), and providers and clients describe obstacles and supports for their attainment of their vision. The subsequent plan either mitigates obstacles or augments supports. When a provider is not sure where to intervene, obstacles to success are often efficient leverage points (see **Fig. 1** for an example of this, regarding case 2).

SUMMARY

Family therapy is a powerful and underused modality for addressing problems faced by children with ASD and their families. Following a nonlinear, patient-centered model, family therapy interventions seek to reorganize family structures and narratives to create new meanings and understandings in the systems that surround and include children with ASD. Families of children with ASD face multiple challenges, including the loss of the imagined child, the weight of a disorder without clear cause, the intense demands of raising a child with special needs, and the comorbid psychiatric and behavioral symptoms that may accompany ASD.

Therapists can play a crucial role in assisting families and children in addressing grief; clearing developmental hurdles; expectation matching; freeing the children as the symptom-bearers; and forming new, more positive family narratives, among other tasks. A family therapist is also ideally positioned to help families refocus on strengths and possibilities as they travel through the often deficit-focused and symptom-focused medical system. Multiple schools of family therapy theory may be applied to this population, with strategic, narrative, and structural interventions offering approaches that may be particularly suited for the challenges typically faced by children with ASD and their families. Although family therapy, like other therapies, offers no cure for ASD, attuned therapists can play a critical role in helping families and children to develop meaning in the lives they have, acceptance of those they do not, and thereby to function at their fullest capacity.

ACKNOWLEDGMENTS

In the spirit of patient-centered and family-centered care, we asked a parent of a child with ASD, Sandy Sullivan, to participate in the writing of this article. Her expertise and insights were extremely valuable throughout our writing process. In addition, the authors thank Liz Brenner, LICSW, John Sargent, MD; and Corky Becker, PhD; our teachers of family therapy.

REFERENCES

1. Kanner L. Autistic disturbances of affective contact. Nervous Child 1943;2: 217–50.
2. Leeds-Hurwitz W. Social construction of reality. In: Littlejohn S, Foss K, editors. Encyclopedia of communication theory. Thousand Oaks (CA): SAGE Publications; 2009. p. 892–5.

3. American Psychiatric Association. Diagnostic and statistical manual of mental disorders. 5th edition. Arlington (VA): American Psychiatric Publishing; 2013.
4. Joshi G, Petty C, Wozniak J, et al. The heavy burden of psychiatric comorbidity in youth with autism spectrum disorders: a large comparative study of psychiatrically referred population. J Autism Dev Disord 2010;40:1361–70.
5. Simonoff E, Pickles A, Charman T, et al. Psychiatric disorders in children with autism spectrum disorders: prevalence, comorbidity, and associated factors in a population-derived sample. J Am Acad Child Adolesc Psychiatry 2008;47:921–9.
6. Levy SE, Giarelli E, Lee L, et al. Autism spectrum disorder and co-occurring developmental, psychiatric, and medical conditions among children in multiple populations of the United States. J Dev Behav Pediatr 2010;31:267–75.
7. Volkmar F, Cook EH Jr, Pomeroy J, et al. Practice parameters for the assessment and treatment of children, adolescents, and adults with autism and other pervasive developmental disorders. J Am Acad Child Adolesc Psychiatry 1999;38: 32S–54S.
8. LoVullo SV, Matson JL. Comorbid psychopathology in adults with autism spectrum disorders and intellectual disabilities. Res Dev Disabil 2009;30:1288–96.
9. Levy A, Perry A. Outcomes in adolescents and adults with autism: a review of the literature. Res Autism Spectr Disord 2011;5:1271–82.
10. Ikeda E, Hinckson E, Krägeloh C. Assessment of quality of life in children and youth with autism spectrum disorder: a critical review. Qual Life Res 2014;23: 1069–85.
11. Volkmar F, Siegel M, Woodbury-Smith M, et al. Practice parameter for the assessment and treatment of children and adolescents with autism spectrum disorder. J Am Acad Child Adolesc Psychiatry 2014;53:237–57.
12. Fisher WW, Groff RA, Roane HS. Applied behavioral analysis: history, philosophy, principles, and basic methods. In: Fisher WW, Piazza CC, Roane HS, editors. Handbook of applied behavioral analysis. New York: The Guilford Press; 2011. p. 3–16.
13. Dawson G, Rogers S, Munson J, et al. Randomized, controlled trial of an intervention for toddlers with autism: the Early Start Denver Model. Pediatrics 2010;125: e17–23.
14. Verschuur R, Didden R, Lang R, et al. Pivotal response treatment for children with autism spectrum disorders: a systematic review. Journal of Autism and Developmental Disorders 2014;1:34–61.
15. Rao PA, Beidel DC, Murray MJ. Social skills interventions for children with Asperger's syndrome or high-functioning autism: a review and recommendations. J Autism Dev Disord 2008;38:353–61.
16. Mailloux Z, Mulligan S, Roley SS, et al. Verification and clarification of patterns of sensory integrative dysfunction. Am J Occup Ther 2011;65:143–51.
17. Lerna A, Esposito D, Conson M, et al. Long-term effects of PECS on social-communication skills of children with autism spectrum disorders: a follow-up study. Int J Lang Commun Disord 2014;49:478–85.
18. Liptak GS, Stuart T, Auinger EP. Health care utilization and expenditures for children with autism: data from U.S. national samples. J Autism Dev Disord 2006;36:871–9.
19. Wagner DV, Borduin CM, Kanne SM, et al. Multisystemic therapy for disruptive behavior problems in youths with autism spectrum disorders: a progress report. J Marital Fam Ther 2014;40:319–31.
20. Jarbrink K, Fombonne E, Knapp M. Measuring the parental, service and cost impacts of children with autistic spectrum disorder: a pilot study. J Autism Dev Disord 2003;33:395–402.

21. Sawyer MG, Bittman M, La Greca AM, et al. Time demands of caring for children with autism: what are the implications for maternal mental health? J Autism Dev Disord 2010;40:620–8.
22. Montes G, Halterman JS. Association of childhood autism spectrum disorders and loss of family income. Pediatrics 2008;121:e821–6.
23. Montes G, Halterman JS. Child care problems and employment among families with preschool-aged children with autism in the United States. Pediatrics 2008; 122:e202–8.
24. Schieve LA, Boulet SL, Kogan MD, et al. Parenting aggravation and autism spectrum disorder: 2007 National Survey of Children's Health. Disabil Health 2011;4: 143–52.
25. Zablotsky B, Bradshaw CP, Stuart EA. The association between mental health, stress, and coping supports in mothers of children with autism spectrum disorder. J Autism Dev Disord 2013;43:1380–93.
26. Benson PR, Kersh J. Marital quality and psychological adjustment among mothers of children with ASD: cross-sectional and longitudinal relationships. J Autism Dev Disord 2011;41:1675–85.
27. Higgins DJ, Bailey SR, Pearce JC. Factors associated with functioning style and coping strategies of families with a child with an autism spectrum disorder. Autism 2005;9:125–37.
28. Hartley SL, Barker ET, Seltzer MM, et al. The relative risk and timing of divorce in families of children with an autism spectrum disorder. J Fam Psychol 2010;24: 449–57.
29. Green L. The well-being of siblings of individuals with autism. ISRN Neurol 2013; 2013:1–7.
30. Woodgate RL, Ateah C, Secco L. Living in a world of our own: the experience of parents who have a child with autism. Qual Health Res 2008;18:1075–83.
31. Madanes C. Strategic family therapy. San Francisco (CA): Jossey-Bass; 1981.
32. Weingarten K. Making sense of illness narratives: braiding theory, practice, and the embodied life. In: White C, editor. Working with the stories of women's lives. Adelaide (South Australia): Dulwich Centre Publications; 2001.
33. Bowen M. Family therapy in clinical practice. New York: Jason Aronson; 1978.
34. Minuchin S. Families and family therapy. Cambridge (MA): Harvard University Press; 1974.
35. White M, Epston D. Narrative means to therapeutic ends. New York: WW Norton; 1990.
36. Cashin A. Narrative therapy: a psychotherapeutic approach in the treatment of adolescents with Asperger's disorder. J Child Adolesc Psychiatr Nurs 2008;21: 48–56.
37. Tomm K. Externalizing the problem and internalizing personal agency. Journal of Strategic and Systemic Therapies 1989;8:1–5.
38. White M. Re-authoring lives: interview & essays. Adelaide (South Australia): Dulwich Centre Publications; 1995.
39. McDaniel SH, Hepworth J, Doherty WJ. Medical family therapy: a biopsychosocial approach to families with health problems. New York: Basic Books; 1992.
40. Madsen WC. Collaborative therapy with multi-stressed families. 2nd edition. New York: The Guildford Press; 2007.

Brief Family-Based Intervention for Substance Abusing Adolescents

Lynn Hernandez, PhD[a],*, Ana Maria Rodriguez, MS[a],
Anthony Spirito, PhD, ABPP[b]

KEYWORDS

- Adolescence • Substance use • Parenting • Family interventions

KEY POINTS

- Parenting plays a key role in an adolescent's use of substances.
- Parental monitoring, consistent limit setting, and parent–child communication about and disapproval of substance use are strategies to protect against adolescent substance misuse and problems.
- Brief parent-focused interventions that support use of these parenting strategies can play an important role in the prevention of adolescent substance use problems.
- The Family Check-up is an example of such a brief intervention.

This article describes a brief intervention designed to improve parenting strategies because of their important role in the onset and escalation of adolescent substance use.[1-3] Alcohol and other drug use are initiated typically during adolescence and escalate over this developmental period. This pattern is so common that some describe substance use disorders (SUD) as "developmental disorders."[4] Nationally representative data demonstrate that approximately 27.8% of adolescents have experimented with alcohol and 16.4% have experimented with marijuana by the time they reach the eighth grade and that these rates increase to 68.2% and 45.5%, respectively, by the time adolescents reach the twelfth grade.[5] Data on levels of problematic drinking, from being drunk to binge drinking also demonstrate important age-related patterns. For example, 12.2% of eighth-grade adolescents reported ever being drunk and 5.1% reported binge drinking (defined as ≥ 5 drinks on 1 occasion) in the past 2 weeks. By the time these adolescents reach the twelfth grade, their rates of ever

The authors have nothing to disclose.
[a] Center for Alcohol and Addiction Studies, Brown University School of Public Health, Box G-S121-5, Providence, RI 02912, USA; [b] Department of Psychiatry and Human Behavior, Alpert Medical School of Brown University, Box G-BH, Providence, RI, 02912, USA
* Corresponding author. Department of Behavioral and Social Sciences, Center for Alcohol and Addiction Studies, Brown University School of Public Health, Box G-S121-5, Providence, RI 02912.
E-mail address: Lynn_Hernandez@Brown.edu

Child Adolesc Psychiatric Clin N Am 24 (2015) 585–599
http://dx.doi.org/10.1016/j.chc.2015.02.010
1056-4993/15/$ – see front matter © 2015 Elsevier Inc. All rights reserved.

childpsych.theclinics.com

Abbreviations	
ATP	Adolescent Transitions Program
FAsTask	Family Assessment Task
FCU	Family Check-up
MDFT	Multidimensional family therapy
MI	Motivational interviewing
MST	Multisystemic therapy
SUD	Substance use disorders

being drunk increase to 52.3% and their rates of binge drinking in the past 2 weeks increase to 23.7%.[5]

Despite these data demonstrating that experimentation with alcohol and marijuana during adolescence is a developmentally normative behavior, research has demonstrated that the earlier a person initiates alcohol and other drug use, the greater their risk for developing a SUD later in life.[6] Underage drinking and early drug use are also associated with a wide range of problems including co-occurring mental health problems (eg, attention deficit hyperactivity disorder, conduct disorder, depression, anxiety), academic problems including school drop-out, delinquent behaviors, and injuries and motor vehicle crashes.[7] For example, in the United States alone, about one-third of 15- to 20-year-olds who died in motor vehicle crashes in 2011 had consumed alcohol.[8] Furthermore, use of alcohol and drugs is also linked to sexual risk taking, including unplanned sexual intercourse, sex without a condom, sex with someone whose sexually transmitted infection status is unknown, and sex with multiple partners.[9] Studies have demonstrated that alcohol use doubles the risk of adolescents engaging in behaviors risky for contracting the human immunodeficiency virus, and that the association between alcohol use and unprotected vaginal intercourse is almost 4 times higher among alcohol users than nonusers.[10] As for marijuana users, they are almost 5 times more likely to have unprotected vaginal intercourse than adolescents who do not use marijuana.[10] The risk of sexual victimization is also greater on days when adolescents drink than on days when they do not drink,[11] and this risk increases with adolescents' level of blood alcohol concentration.[12]

Health problems specific to marijuana use include aggravation of asthma, bronchitis, and emphysema. Chronic use may cause functional alterations in the respiratory system and produce morphologic changes in the airways that precede lung and bronchial cancer.[13] Further, long-term marijuana smokers show cognitive impairment,[14] and early onset of marijuana use (before age 16) has been associated with chronic deficit in attention skills.[15] For example, in the Dunedin study where 1037 individuals between the ages of 7 and 13 who had not initiated marijuana use were administered cognitive tests and then followed into middle adulthood,[16] those who met criteria for cannabis use disorder at 3 or more of the follow-up assessments as adolescents had a 6-point lower full scale IQ score than those who met diagnostic criteria for a cannabis used disorder as adults. These findings suggest that the onset of heavy marijuana use in adolescence, rather than adulthood, can result in long-term cognitive effects. Findings such as these not only indicate that adolescent substance use is a public health concern, but they also underscore the importance of intervening on substance abuse during adolescence.

DIAGNOSING SUBSTANCE-RELATED DISORDERS

There are numerous substances for which a diagnosis of a SUD can be reached, including alcohol, cannabis, hallucinogens, inhalants, opioids, sedatives/hypnotics/

anxiolytics, stimulants, and tobacco. The publication of the fifth edition of the *Diagnostic and Statistical Manual of Mental Disorders*[17] was notable for its elimination of substance abuse and dependence as distinct disorders. In this fifth edition, a single diagnosis of substance use disorder may be obtained if an individual exhibits at least 2 symptoms across domains within a year period. The severity of the disorder, that is, mild (eg, 2–3 symptoms are present), moderate (eg, 4–5 symptoms are present), or severe (eg, ≥6 symptoms are present) is then indicated. These symptoms can span 1 or more domains. The first domain is composed of loss-of-control behaviors, such as frequent overuse of the substance. Social difficulties resulting from substance use is the second domain and includes persistent interpersonal problems caused by or exacerbated by the substance. Risky behavior, such as continuing to use a substance despite recurrent physical or psychological problems, is the third domain. The final domain refers to physiologic changes that result from use of a substance, such as the need to use greater amounts to achieve the same effects as once experienced, tolerance, craving, and withdrawal. When assessing for symptoms within this domain, however, clinicians should remain cognizant that physiologic symptoms, such as tolerance, may be developmentally normative for adolescents and young adults as they move from experimental use to regular use, and that symptoms such as withdrawal and craving are less well-understood in adolescence. Further clarification as to how these symptoms manifest during this developmental stage is needed.[18]

FAMILY FACTORS AFFECTING ADOLESCENT SUBSTANCE USE

There are a number of risk and protective factors that influence alcohol and other drug use behaviors among adolescents. Contextual factors reflect the social ecology of human development and focus on the interconnections among various sources of risk and protection in adolescents' lives.[19] Within this theoretic framework, the family is the most influential microsystem of adolescent development.[20] Risk and protective processes related to alcohol and other drug use within this microsystem include parent–adolescent communication,[2] monitoring and supervision,[21] parental involvement in adolescents' activities and peer relationships,[22] general family management strategies,[1] and parent disapproval and modeling.[23]

When it comes to family management and its effect on adolescent development, parental monitoring and knowledge are perhaps the 2 variables with the most empirical evidence.[24] Parental monitoring can be defined as "a set of correlated parenting behaviors involving attention to and tracking of the adolescent's whereabouts, activities, and adaptations."[25] This definition implies an intentional aspect whereby parents actively seek information regarding their adolescent's behavior.[24] Parental knowledge represents the result of monitoring behaviors and other information acquisition methods like child disclosure.[26] Research has consistently shown that a low level of parental monitoring is related to early use of alcohol and drugs.[21]

Whereas parental monitoring has been identified in the literature as a protective factor for adolescent substance use, affiliation with substance-using peers is a risk factor.[27] Early studies examining the effects of parental monitoring on adolescent substance use after controlling for peer use have produced divergent results. For instance, in studies where peer-related variables and family factors were both evaluated, some research has shown that peer associations have a more profound impact on substance use than parent–adolescent relationships.[28] Others, in contrast, have found that parents exert more influence over adolescent substance use initiation.[27] Research has also demonstrated that these 2 contextual variables affect each other and likely interact to predict adolescent use.[29] As a result, more accepted models of risk now examine parental monitoring as mediators and moderators of adolescent substance use. Such models demonstrate that inadequate parental monitoring increases the risk of adolescent substance use because it allows the adolescent to associate with deviant peers,[30] whereas models of moderation demonstrate that a peer's influence on an adolescent's substance use behavior varies according to the level of parental monitoring the adolescent experiences.[31] One study by Nash and colleagues[32] found that positive parenting was linked with adolescents' strong sense of self-efficacy in refusing peer alcohol offers, thus demonstrating the mechanisms by which parental monitoring can protect adolescents from the negative effects of deviant peer influences.

Parent alcoholism and a family history of alcoholism has been suggested as leading to increased adolescent alcohol use through negative pathways, such as decreased parental monitoring of alcohol use.[33,34] A study with 4731 teens found parental alcohol use to be associated positively with teens' substance-related behaviors, and that these associations were mediated by teens' perceptions of parenting practices, especially among the younger teens. Furthermore, perceived parental monitoring and discipline had unique mediating effects on adolescents' drinking.

Positive parent–teen affective quality, including parent–teen communication, also have important protective influences on teen substance use.[35] However, it is not just positive communication that deters adolescents from substance, use but also the content, style, and timing of communication about use.[36] For instance, Cohen and associates[37] found that children's risk for tobacco onset and alcohol use in the past month was associated with the amount of time children reported their parents spent with them as well as the frequency of communication. Ackard and colleagues[38] found that both male and female adolescents who perceived difficulty in talking to their parents about substance use and related problems were at increased risk for substance use. Consistent with these findings, enhancing the frequency and quality of parent–child communication is a common target in substance use interventions for adolescents.[39]

Strong parental norms against teenage drinking and communication of parental disapproval of drinking have also been shown to reduce the risk of initiation in early adolescence[40] and have been linked to less peer influence to use alcohol, greater self-efficacy to refuse alcohol, and lower frequency of alcohol use behavior.[32] Similarly, national data demonstrate that adolescents who believe that their parents would strongly disapprove of them using substances are significantly less likely to use that substance than adolescents whose parents only somewhat disapproved.[41] Further, communication of alcohol-specific rules in a clear and strict manner is associated with the postponement of drinking in both younger and older adolescents.[42] Other studies, however, have shown that younger adolescents are more strongly affected by the attitudes of their parents,[43] suggesting the need to intervene early on.

In summary, research has shown consistently that a lack of parental involvement in the activities of their children predicts initiation of substance use. Parental monitoring, as well as youth disclosure about their whereabouts and peer affiliations,[26] is related to lower rates of substance use,[44] and regular parent–child communication about substance use as well as parents' disapproval of substance use reduces the risk of early onset substance use. Taken together, this evidence suggests that affecting family processes is critically important in reducing substance misuse during adolescence. Therefore, programs that promote parenting behavior management skills, strengthen parent–child relationships, and work directly with parents by strengthening their sense of responsibility and control over their adolescents' lives can be efficacious at reducing risk for substance use in early adolescence.[45]

FAMILY-BASED INTERVENTIONS

Reviews of prevention programs indicate that active parent participation is a key element in effective substance use programming with children and adolescents,[46] especially when considering longer term outcomes (>3 years).[47] Based on a review of the literature on drug and alcohol prevention programs, for example, Cuijpers[46] concluded that working solely with the child is not likely to result in strong, positive changes in behavior, although it may affect knowledge. In another review, Cowan and Cowan[48] provide further evidence that parents have effects on youth in the family, at school, and within their peer groups, and that family-focused interventions can effect positive changes on child development. Lochman and van den Steenhoven[49] also report multiple positive effects for parent training and family skill building prevention programs, including decreased child problem behaviors, increased prosocial behaviors, decreased substance use, and improved family relations and parenting practices.

Given the empirical evidence reviewed thus far, it is no wonder that family and parenting approaches to prevention and intervention of adolescent substance misuse have received widespread support in the literature.[50] In 1 review,[51] family therapy was compared with family education, individual tracking through schools/courts, and individual and group therapy. Family therapy resulted in greater reductions in substance use in 7 of 8 studies.[51] Furthermore, after reviewing family-based interventions for adolescent substance use, Kumpfer and assocaites[52] concluded that family-based interventions have average effect sizes 2 to 9 times larger than adolescent-only programs. A more recent review by Becker and Curry[50] found ecological family therapy (ie, multisystemic therapy [MST], multidimensional family therapy [MDFT], family systems network, ecologically based family therapy) to be the most evaluated therapy of adolescent outpatient substance abuse treatment. Of the 7 studies on ecological family therapy, 3 demonstrated superior outcomes to other active treatment conditions. Three other studies found ecological family therapy models to have comparable outcomes to usual care in the community as well as cognitive–behavioral therapy and motivational enhancement therapy.

Ecological family therapy approaches attempt to achieve their outcomes by involving parents as essential participants in treatment. The most common ecological family therapy approaches include brief strategic family therapy,[53] family behavior therapy,[54] functional family therapy,[55] MDFT,[56] and MST.[57] Ecological family therapy attempts to restructure family interaction patterns that may be increasing risk for or sustaining an adolescent's substance use behaviors, while also applying behavioral approaches of operant and social learning theories within the family context to promote prosocial behaviors and reduce substance abuse.[50] Often, these approaches extend beyond the family and target all aspects of an adolescents' social context. For example, in MDFT, individuals and systems that intersect to exert a meaningful influence in the adolescent's life are included in treatment (see "Multisystemic Treatment for Externalizing Disorders" by Zajac elsewhere in this issue for more on MDFT).[56]

The majority of treatment studies published have been conducted with adolescents with substance abuse or dependence diagnoses rather than with adolescents in the earlier stages of substance use. Therefore, engaging families in programs targeting substance use remains a significant obstacle to the implementation of successful prevention and intervention programs.[58] Parent interventions usually suffer from low attendance and low retention rates.[59] Low attendance rates can be the result of busy work schedules and extracurricular activity schedules for youth, as well as a lack of motivation. For families whose teens are in the earlier stages of substance use and are perhaps not seeking intensive treatment programs, brief interventions may be the most appropriate and most engaging.

Brief interventions can be described as targeted, time-limited, and low-threshold services that aim to reduce substance use and its associated risks, as well as prevent progression to more severe levels of use.[60] With the exception of 1 intervention, the Family Check-Up (FCU), very few family-based interventions for adolescent substance use meet these criteria. The FCU is a brief assessment and feedback intervention, based on motivational interviewing (MI) principles, that is designed to enhance parental recognition of child risk behaviors and motivation for reducing these problem behaviors and associated risk factors. Metzler and colleagues[61] reviewed 11 best practice lists and identified 9 evidence-based adolescent programs that focused on prevention or treatment of substance use. Five were treatment programs (eg, Strengthening Families[62]), 3 were universal prevention programs (eg, Strengthening Families[63]), but only one was an indicated prevention program, the Adolescent Transitions Program (ATP[64]). The FCU is the primary intervention component of the ATP.

THE FAMILY CHECKUP

The FCU includes techniques endorsed by researchers in the field of family-based preventive interventions,[65] including focusing on protective factors in the family, that is, parental strengths and competencies, presenting normative developmental guidelines, intervening in both parenting practices and family process characteristics, using skills-oriented rather than educational interventions, and attending to the psychosocial issues of the parents. The FCU intervention targets specific family risk and protective factors linked to substance use, including parental supervision and monitoring[25] and parent–child relationship quality.[66] By providing individualized feedback, and using MI techniques, the FCU is designed to motivate families to take action to change current practices when necessary.

There are several studies supporting the efficacy of the FCU (**Table 1**). In an initial efficacy study, Dishion and co-workers[67] found that the FCU reduced the risk for future substance use (measured in the ninth grade) among sixth-grade students (n = 71) from 3 multiethnic urban middle schools. Further, parents assigned to the FCU maintained monitoring practices in the first year of high school, and analyses showed that the prevention effect of the FCU was mediated by changes in parental monitoring. By the 3-year follow-up (first year of high school for adolescents), whereas control group families reduced their monitoring practices, intervention families maintained parental monitoring of youth.[67] These findings point to the prevention effect of the FCU on substance use as mediated by parental monitoring. Thus, conducting MI with parents may influence indirectly behavioral changes among adolescent offspring by improving parenting practices.

The FCU has also been used to specifically address adolescent alcohol misuse.[68] In 1 study, families of adolescents (ages 13–17) who were treated in an urban hospital emergency department for an alcohol-related event were randomized to receive either an individual MI with the teen only or the individual MI plus the FCU. Results demonstrated reductions in quantity of drinking at 3, 6, and 12 months of follow-up, with the strongest effects at 3 and 6 months. The FCU in combination with the MI, however, was found to be superior to individual MI alone in reducing the frequency of high-volume drinking at 6 months after the intervention. This study demonstrated the added benefit of including a parent-based MI in reducing adolescents' drinking.

Conducting a family checkup session

Dishion and Kavanagh[64] developed the FCU to be conducted with parents of at-risk youth. The FCU, as adapted by Spirito and colleagues[68] to address adolescent substance use, is a 2-session intervention composed of the following: (1) an initial intake interview to identify strengths and challenges and engage the family, as well as a videotaped observational task of family interactional style, and (2) a parent feedback session that uses an MI style to encourage maintenance of current positive parenting practices and changes in parenting problems. The goal of the intervention is to reduce problem behaviors among youth and to increase parental motivation toward constructive parenting. The FCU begins with self-report assessments and a videotaped Family Assessment Task (FAsTask[69]), adapted by Dishion and Kavanagh.[64]

Family Assessment Task

The FAsTask is used to assess parent–teen interactions and provide additional assessment information for feedback in the FCU. A FAsTask specifically designed for substance using teens is as follows:

For 3 minutes: Parents and teen plan an activity (relationship quality).
For 5 minutes: Parents lead a discussion about a teen behavior they would like to increase and how they would encourage the process (encouraging growth).
For 5 minutes: Teen leads a discussion about a time without supervision and parents seek additional information (monitoring).
For 5 minutes: Parents lead a discussion on setting limits over the previous month (limit setting).
For 5 minutes: The entire family discusses a "hot" family problem (problem solving).
For 5 minutes: Parents lead a discussion on the family beliefs about alcohol, marijuana, or other drug use (alcohol and drug use norms).
For 3 minutes: Parents recognize a positive attribute of the teen (positive recognition).

The authors have adapted a structured clinical codebook developed by the creators of the FCU for use with substance using adolescents that includes coding procedures to be completed by 2 independent raters, one of which is the treatment provider. "Macro" clinical scores are calculated and coded as an area of "strength," "needs improvement," or "challenge," and provided as feedback during the FCU session. Macro scores include feedback on positive parent–teen relationships, monitoring, limit setting, problem solving, and alcohol and drug use norms. These data, along with parent self-report measures on monitoring and supervision, parent–child communication, prosocial and deviant peer affiliations, and other measures of limit setting and house rules, are used to generate the individualized feedback report for use in the parent feedback session described next.

The Family Checkup Session

The FCU session is designed to improve both the consistency and quality of communication of parental expectations, supervision, limit setting, and monitoring based on a strong underlying platform of parent–teen communication. There are 4 specific phases of the feedback session in the FCU.

1. *Self-assessment*: Parents are asked what they learned about their family from participating in the FAsTask assessment.
2. *Support and clarification*: The counselor assesses level of understanding and clarifies issues within the family.

Table 1
Randomized family check-up trials for adolescent substance use

Author	Referral Source/Recruitment Site	Sample	N	Treatment and Control Groups	Findings
Spirito et al,[68] 2011	Emergency department	Adolescents aged 13–17 y who tested positive for alcohol	125	IMI + FCU IMI	Both conditions reported reductions in substance use at 3 and 6 mo follow-up. Participants in the IMI + FCU conditions reported a larger reduction in high volume drinking days at 6-mo follow-up compared with IMI only.
Stormshak et al,[70] 2004	Middle school	sixth grade, high-risk adolescents and their families	593	FCU Regular school services	FCU led to lower levels of substance use and antisocial behaviors over time compared with treatment as usual.
Connell et al,[71] 2007	Middle schools	Adolescents aged 11–17 y and their families	998	Sixth graders assigned to family-centered intervention and offered a multilevel intervention that includes: 1. Universal classroom-based intervention 2. FCU (offered to high-risk families identified by teachers) 3. Family management treatment	Adolescents whose parents completed the FCU exhibited less growth in alcohol, tobacco, and marijuana use and problem behavior from ages 11 to 17 and lower risk for substance use diagnoses and police arrest records by age 18.

| Dishion and Kavanagh,[64] 2003 | Public middle school; referred by teachers | Sixth- and 7th-grade high-risk adolescents and their families | 71 | FCU Family-centered intervention | Parental monitoring mediated substance use among high-risk adolescents. Parents in the comparison condition reduced their supervision and monitoring between 7th and ninth grades, increasing adolescent substance use over time. Parents completing the FCU reduced supervision and monitoring between 7th and eighth grades but increased between eighth and ninth grades, resulting in less adolescent substance use by ninth grade. |

Abbreviations: FCU, family checkup; IMI, individual motivational interviewing.

3. *Feedback*: This section covers personalized feedback on 3 specific areas of family functioning: expectations regarding substance use, monitoring, and parent–teen communication.
4. *Parenting plan*: The session concludes with a discussion of the teen's strengths and the importance of praising good behavior. Throughout the session, the counselor works with the parent to develop a brief, written Action Plan about communication and monitoring.

Parent motivation for change, change options, and specific steps for making positive changes in parenting are discussed, including barriers to change and foreseeable benefits of change to parents. Positive aspects of parenting are emphasized to instill confidence and to encourage open communication. Tips on "talking to your teen without it being a turn-off," which include the use of "*I* messages" and active listening, are reviewed. Further, examples of common parenting situations (eg, obeying curfews) are used to discuss key parenting practices and the importance of generating plans to deal with these situations. Information on how to monitor teens, especially with respect to substance use is presented using the 5 *W*s worksheet (*W*ho, *W*hat, *W*here, *W*hen, and *W*hy). Peers and siblings are discussed as potential negative influences on teen substance use that need to be addressed when considering parent monitoring strategies.

CASE EXAMPLE

We present a snapshot of the FCU involving a 17-year-old girl referred by Truancy Court for skipping school and smoking marijuana. In this example, the therapist discusses the importance of setting clear limits and being consistent with consequences.

T: I put limit setting between a strength and challenge because in the video you said you have been nagging Emily about hanging out with friends who smoke but you did not do anything about it. Studies have shown that limit setting and consequences are really important in lowering teen substance use. Does limit setting seem to be a challenge for you?

P: She is not very social with her peers, so she is home all the time and I want her to go out. But there is one girl that I do not want her hanging around with because that is who she got in trouble with.

T: I do not know if you remember her comment that she never knows if it is okay for her to be out with certain friends or when she needs to be in by.

P: I tell her when she needs to be in. I could talk to her till I am blue in the face. I think some of that is making excuses. And it is mainly that one girl but I also do not want her to stay inside all the time.

T: So you have mixed feelings about this. But I wonder if there is any consequence for not obeying a rule.

P: That is where I fall short because it seems important but not that important.

T: So she knows if she does not obey your rule, nothing will happen.

P: I guess I just do not know how to punish her at her age.

T: The reason I bring it up is because on the tape it seems like there was some conflict over that. We know that a parenting style of warmth, democracy, and control seems best with respect to limiting adolescents' behavior problems.

ADDITIONAL CONSIDERATIONS

The FCU is conducive to addressing the most common issues that therapists encounter whenever working with parents regarding adolescent substance use. First, the FCU's nonjudgmental approach helps to overcome resistance that may be encountered from parents who either do not feel that monitoring and limit setting is necessary with teens or that substance use is not a problem for their teen. Second, given that substance use varies as teens progress through adolescence, recommendations to parents must be sensitive to these developmental periods. For instance, as adolescents seek greater autonomy from their parents, therapists can help parents to develop monitoring and supervision strategies that are congruent with their adolescent's developmental stage (eg, monitoring the adolescent rides vs the adolescent driving). Similarly, the video assessment provides an opportunity for parents to hear if their adolescents' have positive cognitions regarding alcohol and drugs, which tend to increase as adolescents grow older. In addition to supporting plans for parents to address these positive expectancies through their family management skills, therapists may also consider the benefits of addressing intrapersonal factors (ie, attitudes, expectancies, and social norms) at the adolescent individual level. In fact, as evidenced by Spirito and colleagues,[68] the FCU can be delivered easily in conjunction with an adolescent individual intervention.

Further, although the FCU may warrant tailoring to be congruent with a family's cultural background, its emphasis on parenting and family may be particularly useful for individuals from cultures where family plays a central role. For instance, for Hispanics, for whom *familismo* is an integral part of their culture, the FCU may be a particularly relevant approach to dealing with adolescent substance use. The FCU supports parental authority and choice, which is consistent with the structure of Hispanic families and can enhance family adjustment. The FCU's focus on improving parenting self-efficacy may also be particularly useful for immigrant families, because parents may feel they have less control over the lives of their teenagers since arriving in the United States. Finally, given the FCU's self-guided approach, it can be adapted easily to include values, customs, child-rearing traditions, expectancies for child and parent behavior, distinctive stressors, and resources associated with different cultural groups.

SUMMARY

The FCU is a brief, family-based preventive intervention that shows promise for bolstering the key parenting strategies necessary to prevent the onset and escalation of substance misuse in adolescence. Nonetheless, the FCU may be necessary, but not sufficient, to forestall adolescent substance use problems. Other family interventions, such as MDFT and FFT, may be necessary to build on the work begun in the FCU in cases where substance abuse is more severe. Individual adolescent interventions may also be necessary in these cases.

REFERENCES

1. Barnes GM, Farrell MP. Parental support and control as predictors of adolescent drinking, delinquency, and related problem behaviors. J Marriage Fam 1992;54: 763–76.
2. Ellickson PL, Morton SC. Identifying adolescents at risk for hard drug use: racial/ethnic variations. J Adolesc Health 1999;25:382–95.
3. Peterson PL, Hawkins JD, Abbott RD, et al. Disentangling the effects of parental drinking, family management, and parental alcohol norms on current drinking by black and white adolescents. J Res Adoles 1994;4:203–27.
4. Masten AS, Faden VB, Zucker RA, et al. Underage drinking: a developmental framework. Pediatrics 2008;121(Suppl4):S235–51.

5. Johnston LD, O'Malley PM, Miech RA, et al. Monitoring the future national results on drug use: 1975–2013: overview, key findings on adolescent drug use. Ann Arbor (MI): Institute for Social Research, The University of Michigan; 2014.

6. Flory K, Lynam D, Milich R, et al. Early adolescent through young adult alcohol and marijuana use trajectories: early predictors, young adult outcomes, and predictive utility. Dev Psychopathol 2004;16(1):193–213.

7. Hingson R, Kenkel D. Social, health, and economic consequences of underage drinking. In: Bonnie RJ, O'Connell ME, editors. Reducing underage drinking: a collective responsibility. Washington, DC: The National Academies Press; 2004. p. 351–82.

8. National Highway Traffic Safety Administration (NHTSA), Dept. of Transportation (US). Traffic safety facts 2012: Young Drivers. Washington (DC): NHTSA; 2014. Available at: http://www-nrd.nhtsa.dot.gov/Pubs/812019.pdf. Accessed February 18, 2015.

9. Levy S, Sherritt L, Gabrielli J, et al. Screening adolescents for substance use-related high-risk sexual behaviors. J Adolesc Health 2009;45(5):473–7.

10. Thompson RG Jr, Auslander WF. Substance use and mental health problems as predictors of HIV sexual risk behaviors among adolescents in foster care. Health Soc Work 2011;36(1):33–43.

11. Parks KA, Hsieh Y, Bradizza CM, et al. Factors influencing the temporal relationship between alcohol consumption and experiences with aggression among college women. Psychol Addict Behav 2008;22(2):210–8.

12. Neal DJ, Fromme K. Event-level covariation of alcohol intoxication and behavioral risks during the first year of college. J Consult Clin Psychol 2007;75(2):294–306.

13. Hall W, Solowij N, Lemon J. The health and psychological consequences of cannabis use. National drug strategy monograph series no. 25. Canberra (Australia): Australian Government Publishing Service; 1994.

14. Bolla KI, Brown K, Eldreth D, et al. Dose-related neurocognitive effects of marijuana use. Neurology 2002;59(9):1337–43.

15. Pope HG Jr, Yurgelun-Todd D. The residual cognitive effects of heavy marijuana use in college students. JAMA 1996;275(7):521–7.

16. Meier MH, Caspi A, Ambler A, et al. Persistent cannabis users show neuropsychological decline from childhood to midlife. Proc Natl Acad Sci U S A 2012;109(40):E2657–64.

17. American Psychiatric Association. Diagnostic and statistical manual of mental disorders. 5th edition. Washington, DC: American Psychiatric Association; 2013.

18. Winters KC, Martin CS, Chung T. Substance use disorders in DSM-V when applied to adolescents. Addiction 2011;106(5):882–4.

19. Bronfenbrenner U. Contexts of child rearing: problems and prospects. Am Psychol 1979;34(10):844–50.

20. Perrino T, González-Soldevilla A, Pantin H, et al. The role of families in adolescent HIV prevention: a review. Clin Child Fam Psychol Rev 2000;3(2):81–96.

21. Chilcoat HD, Anthony JC. Impact of parent monitoring on initiation of drug use through late childhood. J Am Acad Child Adolesc Psychiatry 1996;35(1):91–100.

22. Hawkins JD, Catalano RF, Miller JY. Risk and protective factors for alcohol and other drug problems in adolescence and early adult- hood: implications for substance abuse prevention. Psychol Bull 1992;112:64–105.

23. Chassin L, Pillow D, Curran P, et al. Relation of parental alcoholism to early adolescent substance use. A test of three mediating mechanisms. J Abnorm Psychol 1993;102:3–19.

24. Crouter AC, Head MR. Parental monitoring and knowledge of children. In: Bornstein MH, editor. Handbook of parenting. 2nd edition. vol. 3. Being and becoming a parent. Mahwah (NJ): Erlbaum; 2002. p. 461–83.
25. Dishion TJ, McMahon RJ. Parental monitoring and the prevention of child and adolescent problem behavior: a conceptual and empirical formulation. Clin Child Fam Psychol Rev 1998;1(1):61–75.
26. Stattin H, Kerr M. Parental monitoring: a reinterpretation. Child Dev 2000;71(4): 1072–85.
27. Wills TA, Resko JA, Ainette MG, et al. Role of parent support and peer support in adolescent substance use: a test of mediated effects. Psychol Addict Behav 2004;18(2):122–34.
28. Beal AC, Ausiello J, Perrin JM. Social influences on health-risk behaviors among minority middle school students. J Adolesc Health 2001;28(6):474–80.
29. Dishion TJ, Nelson SE, Bullock BM. Premature adolescent autonomy: parent disengagement and deviant peer process in the amplification of problem behavior. J Adolesc 2004;27:515–30.
30. Chung HL, Steinberg L. Relations between neighborhood factors, parenting behaviors, peer deviance, and delinquency among serious juvenile offenders. Dev Psychol 2006;42(2):319–31.
31. Kiesner J, Poulin F, Dishion TJ. Adolescent substance use with friends: moderating and mediating effects of parental monitoring and peer activity contexts. Merrill Palmer Q (Wayne State Univ Press) 2010;56(4):529–56.
32. Nash SG, McQueen A, Bray JH. Pathways to adolescent alcohol use: family environment, peer influence, and parental expectations. J Adolesc Health 2005;37(1): 19–28.
33. Latendresse SJ, Rose RJ, Viken RJ, et al. Parenting mechanisms in links between parents' and adolescents' alcohol use behaviors. Alcohol Clin Exp Res 2008; 32(2):322–30.
34. Li C, Pentz MA, Chou CP. Parental substance use as a modifier of adolescent substance use risk. Addiction 2002;97(12):1537–50.
35. Chassin L, Presson CC, Todd M, et al. Maternal socialization of adolescent al transmission of smoking-related beliefs. Dev Psychol 1998;34:1189–201.
36. Jaccard J, Turrisi R. Parent-based intervention strategies to reduce adolescent alcohol-impaired driving. J Stud Alcohol Suppl 1999;13:84–93.
37. Cohen DA, Richardson J, LaBree L. Parenting behaviors and the onset of smoking and alcohol use: a longitudinal study. Pediatrics 1994;94(3):368–75.
38. Ackard DM, Neumark-Sztainer D, Story M, et al. Parent-child connectedness and behavioral and emotional health among adolescents. Am J Prev Med 2006;30(1): 59–66.
39. Beatty SE, Cross DS, Shaw TM. The impact of a parent-directed intervention on parent-child communication about tobacco and alcohol. Drug Alcohol Rev 2008; 27(6):591–601.
40. Kosterman R, Hawkins JD, Guo J, et al. The dynamics of alcohol and marijuana initiation: patterns and predictors of first use in adolescence. Am J Public Health 2000;90(3):360–6.
41. Office of Applied Studies. Results from the 2008 national survey on drug use and health: national findings. Rockville (MD): Substance Abuse and Mental Health Services Administration; 2009.
42. Van Der Vorst H, Engels RC, Deković M, et al. Alcohol-specific rules, personality and adolescents' alcohol use: a longitudinal person-environment study. Addiction 2007;102(7):1064–75.

43. Zhang LN, Welte JW, Wieczorek WF. Peer and parental influences on male adolescent drinking. Subst Use Misuse 1997;32(14):2121–36.
44. Leventhal T, Brooks-Gunn J. The neighborhoods they live in: the effects of neighborhood residence on child and adolescent outcomes. Psychol Bull 2000;126(2): 309–37.
45. Dishion TJ, Andrews DW, Kavanagh K, et al. Preventive interventions for high-risk youth: the Adolescent Transitions Program. In: Peters RD, McMahon RJ, editors. Preventing childhood disorders, AOD abuse, and delinquency. Thousand Oaks (CA): Sage; 1996. p. 184–214.
46. Cuijpers P. Three decades of drug prevention research. Drugs Educ Prev Pol 2003;10(1):7–20.
47. Foxcroft DR, Ireland D, Lister-Sharp DJ, et al. Primary prevention for alcohol misuse in young people. Cochrane Database Syst Rev 2002;(3):CD003024.
48. Cowan PA, Cowan CP. Interventions as tests of family systems theories: marital and family relationships in children's development and psychopathology. Dev Psychopathol 2002;14(4):731–59.
49. Lochman JE, van den Steenhoven A. Family-based approaches to substance abuse prevention. J Prim Prev 2002;23(1):49–114.
50. Becker SJ, Curry JF. Outpatient interventions for adolescent substance abuse: a quality of evidence review. J Consult Clin Psychol 2008;76(4):531–44.
51. Waldron H. Adolescent substance abuse and family therapy outcome. In: Ollendick T, Prinz R, editors. Advances in clinical psychology, vol. 19. New York: Plenum; 1997. p. 199–234.
52. Kumpfer KL, Alvarado R, Whiteside HO. Family-based interventions for substance use and misuse prevention. Subst Use Misuse 2003;38(11–13): 1759–87.
53. Szapocznik J, Scopetta MA, King OE. The effect and degree of treatment comprehensiveness with a Latino drug abusing population. In: Smith DE, Anderson SM, Burton M, et al, editors. A multicultural view of drug abuse. Cambridge (MA): G.K. Hall; 1978. p. 563–73.
54. Azrin N, Donohue B, Besald V, et al. Youth drug abuse treatment: a controlled outcome study. J Child Adolesc Subst Abuse 1994;3:1–16.
55. Barton C, Alexander JF. Functional family therapy. In: Gurman AS, Kniskern DP, editors. Handbook of family therapy. New York: Brunner/Mazel; 1981. p. 403–43.
56. Liddle HA, Hogue A. Multidimensional family therapy for adolescent substance abuse. In: Wagner EF, Waldron HB, editors. Innovations in adolescent substance abuse interventions. Amsterdam (Netherlands): Pergamon/Elsevier Science Inc; 2001. p. 229–61.
57. Henggeler SW, Borduin CM, Melton GB, et al. Effects of multisystemic therapy on drug use and abuse in serious juvenile offenders: a progress report from two outcome studies. Fam Dynam Addiction Q 1991;1(3):40–51.
58. Spoth R, Kavanagh K, Dishion T. Family-centered preventive intervention science: toward benefits to larger populations of children, youth, and families. Prev Sci 2002;3(3):145–52.
59. Goodman MR. If we build it will parents come? Parent participation in preventative parenting groups. Ann Arbor (MI): ProQuest Information & Learning; 2002.
60. Babor TF, McRee BG, Kassebaum PA, et al. Screening, Brief Intervention, and Referral to Treatment (SBIRT): toward a public health approach to the management of substance abuse. Subst Abus 2007;28(3):7–30.
61. Metzler CW, Biglan A, Embry DD, et al. Improving the well-being of adolescents in Oregon. Eugene (OR): Center on Early Adolescence, Oregon Institute; 2007.

62. Liddle HA, Schwartz SJ. Attachment and family therapy: the clinical utility of adolescent-family attachment research. Fam Process 2002;41(3):455–76.
63. Spoth R, Redmond C, Shin C. Direct and indirect latent-variable parenting outcomes of two universal family-focused preventive interventions: extending a public health-oriented research base. J Consult Clin Psychol 1998;66(2):385–99.
64. Dishion TJ, Kavanagh K. Intervening in adolescent problem behavior: a family-centered approach. New York: Guilford Press; 2003.
65. Hogue A, Liddle HA. Family-based preventive intervention: an approach to preventing substance use and antisocial behavior. Am J Orthop 1999;69(3):278–93.
66. Thornberry TP, Huizinga D, Loeber R. The prevention of serious delinquency and violence: implications from the program of research on causes and correlates of delinquency. In: Howell JC, Krisberg B, Hawkins JD, et al, editors. Sourcebook on serious, violent, and chronic juvenile offenders. Thousand Oaks (CA): Sage; 1995. p. 213–37.
67. Dishion TJ, Nelson SE, Kavanagh K. The family check-up with high-risk young adolescents: preventing early-onset substance use by parent monitoring. Behav Ther 2003;34(4):553–71.
68. Spirito A, Sindelar-Manning H, Colby SM, et al. Individual and family motivational interventions for alcohol-positive adolescents treated in an emergency department: results of a randomized clinical trial. Arch Pediatr Adolesc Med 2011; 165(3):269–74.
69. Forgatch MS. Patterns and outcome in family problem-solving - the disrupting effect of negative emotion. J Marriage Fam 1989;51(1):115–24.
70. Stormshak EA, Comeau CA, Shepard SA. The relative contribution of sibling deviance and peer deviance in the prediction of substance use across middle childhood. J Abnorm Child Psychol 2004;32(6):635–49.
71. Connell AM, Dishion TJ, Yasui M, et al. An adaptive approach to family intervention: linking engagement in family-centered intervention to reductions in adolescent problem behavior. J Consult Clin Psychol 2007;75(4):568–79.

Multisystemic Therapy for Externalizing Youth

Kristyn Zajac, PhD*, Jeff Randall, PhD, Cynthia Cupit Swenson, PhD

KEYWORDS

- Multisystemic therapy • Externalizing problems • Substance abuse
- Physical abuse and neglect • Juvenile offenders

KEY POINTS

- Externalizing problems are multidetermined and related to individual, family, peer, school, and community risk factors.
- Multisystemic therapy (MST) is an evidence-based treatment for adolescents with serious clinical problems who are at-risk for out-of-home placement.
- MST targets the multiple determinants of externalizing problems using a home- and community-based intervention model to decrease barriers to service access.
- Adaptations of MST have been shown to be effective for problems related to externalizing behaviors, including substance use and parental physical abuse and neglect.
- Treatment fidelity has been linked to positive outcomes across MST delinquency studies, highlighting the importance of quality assurance through ongoing supervision and support.

Multisystemic therapy (MST) is a family- and community-based intervention originally developed for juvenile offenders.[1] It has since been adapted and evaluated for a range of serious externalizing problems, including violent offending and substance abuse. Of note, some adaptations fall beyond the scope of this review, including MST for psychiatric problems, problem sexual behaviors, and chronic health conditions. The aims of the current article are to describe MST's clinical procedures and

Disclosures: C.C. Swenson is a consultant in the development of MST-CAN programs through MST Services, LLC, which has the exclusive licensing agreement through the Medical University of South Carolina for the dissemination of MST technology. The authors have no other disclosures to report.

This publication was supported by the National Institute on Drug Abuse and the National Institute of Mental Health through Grants K23DA034879 (PI: K. Zajac) and RO1MH60663 (PI: C.C. Swenson).

Department of Psychiatry & Behavioral Sciences, Family Services Research Center, Medical University of South Carolina, 176 Croghan Spur Road, Suite 104, Charleston, SC 29407, USA
* Corresponding author.
E-mail address: zajac@musc.edu

Abbreviations	
CM	Contingency Management
CPS	Child Protective Services
EOT	Enhanced Outpatient Therapy
MST	Multisystemic therapy
MST-BSF	MST-Building Stronger Families
MST-CAN	Multisystemic Therapy for Child Abuse and Neglect
MST-SA	Multisystemic Therapy for Substance Abuse
PTSD	Posttraumatic stress disorder
RCTs	Randomized clinical trials

the substantial support for its effectiveness and provide an overview of 2 adaptations of MST related to externalizing behaviors.

EXTERNALIZING BEHAVIORS: NATURE OF THE PROBLEM

MST targets the types of serious clinical problems that put adolescents at risk for out-of-home placements, including serious externalizing behaviors. Prospective studies have concluded that externalizing behaviors are multidetermined and have identified specific family (eg, parental supervision and skills), school (eg, academic achievement, poor home-school link), peer (eg, deviant peer associations), and neighborhood (eg, high crime rates) factors that increase risk for these behaviors.[2,3] However, before MST, interventions for externalizing youth typically focused on one or a few of these risk factors and produced few positive outcomes. Thus, MST was the first treatment for externalizing problems to use this empirical framework to inform intervention.

MULTISYSTEMIC THERAPY CLINICAL PROCEDURES
Theoretic Underpinnings

MST is based on the theoretic underpinnings of Bronfenbrenner's social ecological framework, which posits that individuals' behaviors are influenced directly and indirectly by the multiple systems in which they are imbedded.[4] Youth are conceptualized as embedded in their family, peer, school, and community systems. In addition, MST recognizes that effects within these systems are reciprocal in nature (eg, youth both are influenced by their peers and have influence on their peer group). Strategic[5] and structural[6] family therapies also inform MST.

Model of Service Delivery

MST uses a home-based model, delivering services where problems occur (ie, homes, schools, and neighborhoods). Such service delivery removes barriers to treatment common to traditional outpatient settings, including transportation problems, lack of childcare, and restricted hours of operation. Furthermore, interacting with families in their homes and communities builds rapport and allows for observation of youth and family behaviors in real-world settings. MST programs include treatment teams, each composed of 3 to 4 Master's-level therapists supervised by a half-time advanced Master's-level or Doctoral-level supervisor. Each therapist carries a caseload of 4 to 6 families, and treatment duration is 4 to 6 months. The MST team is available to families 24 hours per day, 7 days per week through an on-call rotation. This model allows for scheduling appointments at times that are convenient to families, effective crisis management, and high levels of direct service for each family (ie, an average of 60 hours over the course of treatment).

Principles and Analytical Process

MST provides a framework through which treatment occurs, using a set of 9 core principles and a structured analytical process. The 9 principles are presented in **Box 1** and provide the underlying infrastructure that defines the MST model. Adherence to these principles predicts positive clinical outcomes.

The MST Analytical Process (ie, the "Do-Loop") is a structured process that therapists follow to help guide clinical decision-making. Using the Do-Loop, therapists first gather information about the referral behavior and desired outcomes from the youth, family, and other key stakeholders (eg, school personnel, probation officers). Using these multiple perspectives, the therapist and team hypothesize the "fit factors" or the "drivers" of the referral behaviors (ie, which factors in the individual, family, peer, school, and community maintain these behaviors and which will decrease or prevent them). Next, the therapist works with the family to prioritize drivers and develop interventions to target each prioritized driver. Therapists closely monitor

---

Box 1
Multisystemic therapy: 9 core principles

Principle 1: Finding the fit

The primary purpose of assessment is to understand the "fit" between the identified problems and their broader systemic context.

Principle 2: Focusing on positives and strengths

Therapeutic contacts should emphasize the positive and should use systemic strengths as levers for change.

Principle 3: Increasing responsibility

Interventions should be designed to promote responsible behavior and decrease irresponsible behavior among family members.

Principle 4: Present focused, action oriented, and well-defined

Interventions should be present-focused and action-oriented, targeting specific and well-defined problems.

Principle 5: Targeting sequences

Interventions should target sequences of behavior within or between multiple systems that maintain the identified problems.

Principle 6: Developmentally appropriate

Interventions should be developmentally appropriate and fit the developmental needs of the youth.

Principle 7: Continuous effort

Interventions should be designed to require daily or weekly effort by family members.

Principle 8: Evaluation and accountability

Intervention efficacy is evaluated continuously from multiple perspectives with providers assuming accountability for overcoming barriers to successful outcomes.

Principle 9: Generalization

Interventions should be designed to promote treatment generalization and long-term maintenance of therapeutic change by empowering caregivers to address family members' needs across multiple systemic contexts.

the implementation of each intervention and problem-solve any barriers. Finally, the therapist gathers information from the family and other stakeholders about the effectiveness of each intervention. If unsuccessful, the therapist moves back through the Do-Loop and works with the family to develop new hypotheses about referral behaviors and a new set of interventions to try. Thus, MST follows an iterative process that allows for learning about problem behaviors through treatment successes and failures.

Targets of Change and Nature of Interventions

Family risk factors are often central to the conceptualization of problem behaviors, and improved family functioning has been shown to mediate the effects of MST on externalizing behaviors.[7–10] Therefore, caregiver monitoring, supervision, family cohesion and support, and provision of consistent rules and consequences are frequent targets of MST. When addressing these factors, MST therapists must be prepared to overcome barriers such as parental mental health problems, substance abuse, and poor parenting skills, all of which may be included in the ongoing conceptualization of problem behaviors.

In addition to family factors, therapists also coach caregivers to target other key risk factors, including association with deviant peers, lack of prosocial activities, and school disengagement. MST therapists empower caregivers to get involved with their child's peer group and set limits on contact with peers who contribute to externalizing behaviors. Similarly, parents are coached to develop positive relationships with teachers and school administrators, with the goal of promoting home-school communication to facilitate educational success. Finally, individual level factors targeted in MST include, for example, deficits in problem-solving skills.

Interventions are based primarily on evidence-based behavioral, cognitive-behavioral, and family systems approaches. For example, therapists are proficient in strategies used in evidence-based family treatment models, including emphasizing familial strengths rather than deficits and reframing negative behaviors and family interactions to produce therapeutic gains. Similarly, MST therapists use well-validated treatments to target individual drivers. For example, as described in later discussion, Contingency Management (CM), an evidence-based treatment for substance use, is often used. Importantly, interventions used to target individual risk factors are done with caregiver involvement to increase the sustainability of change after treatment is completed.

Multisystemic Therapy Quality Assurance/Quality Improvement

A quality assurance and improvement program is used to support fidelity in MST delivery. The emphasis on quality assurance is informed by multiple studies demonstrating the link between treatment fidelity and clinical outcomes in MST trials.[9,11–14]

Procedures have been developed to ensure proper training and oversight of MST delivery. First, each member of the MST team completes a 5-day orientation to the standard MST model. Team members delivering MST adaptations are required to attend additional training on program-specific features. Teams have both weekly on-site group supervision and phone-based consultation with an MST expert as well as quarterly booster trainings. Finally, treatment and supervisory feedback measures are used to continuously monitor fidelity. For example, the MST Therapist Adherence Measure is conducted monthly by an independent interviewer to gather feedback from parents about therapists' adherence to MST principles, and feedback is provided to the treatment team. Thus, quality assurance is designed to be continuous, allow for provider self-reflection, and prevent provider drift.

CASE VIGNETTE #1: MULTISYSTEMIC THERAPY FOR SERIOUS OFFENDING

Maria (age 15) was recently arrested for grand theft auto. This arrest was Maria's first legal charge, and she was sentenced to probation and treatment. Her probation officer referred the family to MST. Maria's problem behavior, including skipping class, arguing with teachers, hanging out with delinquent peers, staying out late, and breaking rules at home, started a year before the arrest. She had been an honor student, but her grades recently plummeted to failing and she had disconnected from positive friends. Maria lives with 2 aunts and 4 cousins under the age of 6. Maria's parents were killed in an auto accident when she was an infant. Her grandmother raised her until she passed away last year from cancer. Because of Maria's grief over losing her grandmother, her aunts did not feel they could establish rules or discipline her. Their primary method of discipline was yelling, but they did not follow through on threats of consequences. They were very angry and told Maria she was a disappointment to her grandmother.

The MST therapist worked with the family to identify fit factors for the problem behaviors. These factors included no rules at home and no consequences for negative behavior. In fact, when her aunts would yell at Maria over something she did wrong, they would feel bad and buy her expensive clothes and tennis shoes afterward. These deficits in parenting were driven by the grief the family was experiencing over the death of Maria's grandmother. They had little time to prepare for the loss because the diagnosis and illness happened quickly.

Interventions included (1) development and implementation of a behavior plan at home; (2) strengthening the home-school link; (3) working with the aunts to ensure Maria met with her probation officer and completed required community service; (4) re-establishing Maria's prior positive peer relationships and breaking the link with negative peers; and, (5) family therapy to address grief reactions. These interventions and resulting family changes allowed Maria to reconnect with positive peers, return to prior levels of functioning at school, and manage her grief. Family therapy was important because it strengthened the bond between Maria and her aunts. No further arrests occurred.

MULTISYSTEMIC THERAPY ADAPTATIONS RELATED TO EXTERNALIZING PROBLEMS

Standard MST has been adapted to treat youth and families with other serious clinical needs. Two adaptations pertinent to this article are multisystemic therapy for substance abuse (MST-SA[15]) and multisystemic therapy for child abuse and neglect (MST-CAN).[16]

Multisystemic Therapy for Substance Abuse

Although substantial data support the effectiveness of standard MST for delinquent youth with substance use problems, MST-SA was designed specifically for agencies that serve youth presenting with substance use as a primary referral behavior. As with delinquent behaviors, multiple risk factors (ie, individual, family, peer, school, and community) influence adolescent substance use,[17] including family factors, such as supervision, discipline strategies, parental support, and parent-child relationship quality.[18–20] One of the strongest predictors of adolescent substance use is peer substance use.[21,22] Other factors, including parental substance use, exert indirect influences by limiting parents' ability to supervise youth. MST-SA integrates CM, an evidence-based substance abuse intervention, to target risk factors specific to substance use.

Primary goals of multisystemic therapy for substance abuse

The MST-SA therapists' goals are to teach caregivers to: (1) conduct random screens to detect substance use; (2) develop and implement an incentive system that rewards youth for nonsubstance use and removes incentives when youth use substances; and (3) build supportive social networks. MST-SA also teaches both youth and caregivers how to: (1) conduct functional analyses to understand substance use triggers; (2) address triggers; and (3) use effective drug-refusal strategies. The model emphasizes long-term change that families can maintain after treatment ends.

Treatment model

MST-SA's treatment model is largely identical to standard MST (including the use of the analytical process and 9 principles). The following components are used to address substance use specifically:

- Analysis of Antecedents, Behaviors, and Consequences (ie, functional analyses) of drug use are conducted for each instance of substance use or nonuse.
- Therapists and family members develop Family Drug Management Plans to help the youth avoid substance use.
- Drug-refusal skills involving extensive role-play with the youth and family.
- Random urine drug screens and breathalyzers conducted by caregivers (with guidance from therapists) at the frequency required to detect the youth's drug of choice.
- Voucher Systems and Incentives focus on changing the contingencies for substance use (ie, providing rewards for clean screens and withholding incentives for dirty screens). Caregivers take the lead in deciding on rules and incentives.

CASE VIGNETTE #2: MULTISYSTEMIC THERAPY FOR SUBSTANCE ABUSE FOR SUBSTANCE USE

Marvin (age 17) was arrested for marijuana possession. His presenting problems included smoking marijuana laced with cocaine daily; selling illicit drugs; fighting at school; and school expulsion. Fit factors included Marvin's favorable attitudes toward drug use; unlimited free time; a neighborhood that lacked prosocial outlets; and a lack of clear rules and consequences for his behaviors at home. Triggers for substance use include boredom and seeing negative peers. Initial interventions included attempts to increase his mother's skills in monitoring him and setting clear rules and consequences for his behavior. His therapist worked with his mother to develop a voucher and incentive system, and his mother began conducting random urine drug screens. Marvin had dirty screens for several weeks and spent some days in detention. Marvin's mother was facing numerous practical needs (lack of money for food, the family's heat and water had been turned off) that got in the way of her following through with the plan. The MST-SA therapist assisted Marvin's mother to obtain assistance from other family members and use community supports, including a local food bank. Once the practical needs were addressed, Marvin's mother was able to implement the behavior plan consistently. The MST-SA therapist and Marvin's mother also got Marvin involved in prosocial activities with positive peers and taught Marvin drug-refusal skills. Positive clinical outcomes included Marvin having clean drug screens for a year, obtaining a job at a local restaurant, and completing a GED program.

Multisystemic Therapy for Child Abuse and Neglect

MST-CAN was adapted for families who are under the guidance of Child Protective Services (CPS) due to recent physical abuse and/or neglect, or have a target child between the ages of 6 and 17, and the child is either living with the family or there is a plan to reunite rapidly.

Physical abuse and neglect are related to the development of behavioral and mental health problems, such as aggression, anxiety, depression, posttraumatic stress disorder (PTSD), and self-harm.[23-25] Risk for out-of-home placement and reabuse among such children is high. Similar to externalizing behaviors, risk factors for abuse and neglect exist across several systems[26] and include parental mental health or substance use problems[27]; family conflict and interpersonal violence[28]; developmental delays or behavioral problems[29]; and lack of social support and low use of community resources.[30] As in MST, MST-CAN addresses risk factors for abuse or neglect across multiple systems.

Primary goals

MST-CAN aims to prevent out-of-home placements, assure safety, prevent reabuse and neglect, reduce mental health difficulties, and increase social supports. CPS caseworkers have the difficult task of coordinating care between multiple providers (eg, substance use and mental health treatment providers, psychiatrists, parenting classes), monitoring families' progress, and keeping children safe. This job is complicated by high caseloads of families that can be challenging to engage. MST-CAN greatly simplifies the caseworker's task by providing all services, maintaining ongoing communication with CPS, and monitoring safety. In fact, MST-CAN is heavily endorsed by CPS staff specifically related to increased collaboration and positive changes in families' views of CPS.[31]

Treatment model

MST-CAN's service provision characteristics are similar to standard MST, with the addition of a part-time psychiatrist and a bachelor's-level crisis case worker. Treatment focuses primarily on the adults in the family, but addresses problems among children when necessary, with an average of 5 people treated per family. Although interventions are individualized, the model contains research-supported approaches for problems common across families. Components completed with all families include the following:

- Intensive safety planning, including ecological safety assessments, early in treatment with the clinical team and sometimes with CPS (weekly safety assessments for the first month and as needed after that).
- A clarification process in which the parent addresses cognitions about the abuse/neglect, accepts full responsibility, and reads an apology letter during a family meeting.[32]

Treatment strategies used as-needed include the following:

- Functional analysis for physical abuse or ongoing family conflict to understand sequences of events that lead to aggression. Interventions target triggers for aggression to de-escalate children or parents.
- Cognitive-behavioral treatment of anger management when required by the child or parent.[33]
- Behavioral family treatment for communication difficulties and problem-solving.[34]
- Prolonged exposure therapy[35] for parents with PTSD.
- Reinforcement-based therapy[36] for adults for whom substance abuse puts child safety at risk.[37]

CASE VIGNETTE #3: MULTISYSTEMIC THERAPY FOR CHILD ABUSE AND NEGLECT FOR CHILDHOOD NEGLECT

Jamilla (age 13) and her family were referred by CPS following a substantiated report of neglect. Jamilla missed 50 school days last year and 25 this year so far. When she did attend, she appeared disheveled and often slept in class. Jamilla lives with Ms Ward, her mother, and 2 siblings, ages 4 and 5. She must often care for her siblings due to Ms Ward's substance use (alcohol and cocaine). Ms Ward's mother and siblings currently use drugs and are not available to help. Jamilla's father was imprisoned 2 years ago on drug-related charges and has a 15-year sentence. His family is drug-free and available to help, but Ms Ward is hesitant, because she feels they are judgmental toward her. Interactions between Jamilla and her mother are characterized by arguing and name calling. CPS would like Ms Ward to stop using drugs and alcohol and monitor her children, and Jamilla to attend school 100% of the time.

The target behavior identified by the MST team, CPS, and Jamila's mother was her school nonattendance. The drivers or fit factors included individual (inability to get up in the morning and get ready; depression; anger); parent (drug and alcohol use; low monitoring and supervision; PTSD from a history of sexual abuse as well as physical abuse from her boyfriend who left the home 6 months ago; low parenting skills); school (low connection with school; weak parent-school link); and family (conflicted interactions; poor communication and problem-solving skills).

Based on the assessment of fit factors, the primary drivers of Jamilla's truancy are her mother's weak parenting skills, conflicted interactions between mother and daughter, and weak home-school link. Research-supported interventions were applied to these drivers. Specifically, Ms Ward's parenting skills were low primarily because of her anxiety (PTSD) and substance use. To address these critical problems, Prolonged Exposure therapy was used to treat PTSD and Reinforcement-based therapy was used to treat substance abuse. To improve the home-school link, the therapist worked with Ms Ward and the school to involve Jamilla in school activities and to provide tutoring to help her catch up. Jamilla and her mother's low communication and problem-solving skills prevented them from prioritizing school and developing strategies for attendance. A behavioral family intervention to teach and coach communication and problem-solving skills was used. Finally, family therapy was conducted to reconnect Ms Ward and her children with the father's family, which improved social supports and reduced family stress.

EMPIRICAL SUPPORT FOR MULTISYSTEMIC THERAPY AND ITS ADAPTATIONS

Table 1 summarizes studies evaluating the efficacy and effectiveness of MST, MST-SA, and MST-CAN. For the sake of space, studies solely focusing on mechanisms of action, implementation, or other MST adaptations are not discussed. Additional information on these topics can be found at http://mstservices.com/outcomestudies.pdf.

Standard Multisystemic Therapy

MST is one of only 3 programs for the treatment of delinquency that meets the rigorous Blueprints standards for model programs,[38] which include well-specified treatment protocols, high-quality evaluations demonstrating reduced offending for at least 12 months postintervention, and readiness for transport to community settings. In sum, there have been 18 studies of MST for serious juvenile offenders, including 11 randomized trials, 4 independent studies, 2 international studies, and 1 trial with ultra-long follow-up.[39] There have also been 8 studies with adolescents who have serious conduct problems (but not justice system involvement), including 4 randomized trials, 7 independent evaluations, and 5 international studies. Among serious juvenile offenders across studies, the median reduction in rearrest rates and out-of-home placements has been 42% and 54%, respectively. In addition, multiple studies have shown improved family functioning, decreased substance use and mental health problems,

Table 1
Summary of multisystemic therapy outcome studies

Study	Sample	Design	Findings	Provider/Setting	MST Type
Henggeler et al,[46] 1986	Delinquents (N = 80)	Quasi-experimental; posttreatment evaluations; compared with diversion services	Improved family relations; decreased behavioral problems and association with deviant peers	Graduate students/ university	Standard
Henggeler et al,[47] 1992; Henggeler et al,[48] 1993	Violent and chronic juvenile offenders (N = 84)	RCT; 59-wk and 2.4-y follow-up; compared with usual community services	At 59-wk follow-up: improved family relations; decreased recidivism, and out-of-home placement At 2.4-y follow-up: decreased recidivism	Community therapists/ community provider	Standard
Borduin et al,[49] 1995; Schaeffer & Borduin,[50] 2005; Sawyer & Borduin,[40] 2011	Violent and chronic juvenile offenders (N = 176)	RCT; 4-y, 13.7-y, and 21.9-y follow-ups; compared with individual counseling	At 4-y follow-up: improved family relations, decreased parental psychiatric problems, youth behavior problems, and recidivism At 13.7-y follow-up: decreased rearrests and days incarcerated At 21.9-y follow-up: decreased felony arrests and days in adult confinement	Graduate students/ university	Standard
Henggeler et al,[11] 1997	Violent and chronic juvenile offenders (N = 155)	RCT; 1.7-y follow-up; compared with juvenile probation services	Decreased psychiatric symptoms, incarceration, recidivism; treatment adherence was related to recidivism outcomes	Community therapists/ community providers (2 sites)	Standard

(continued on next page)

Table 1
(continued)

Study	Sample	Design	Findings	Provider/Setting	MST Type
Ogden & Halliday-Boykins,[51] 2004; Ogden & Hagen,[52] 2006	Norwegian youth with serious antisocial behavior (N = 100)	RCT; 6- and 24-mo postrecruitment follow-ups; compared with usual child welfare services	At 6-mo follow-up: decreased externalizing and internalizing symptoms, out-of-home placements, increased social competence, consumer satisfaction. At 24-mo follow-up: decreased internalizing symptoms and out-of-home placements	Community therapists/ community providers	Standard
Timmons-Mitchell et al,[53] 2006	Juvenile offenders (felons) at imminent risk of placement (N = 93)	RCT; 18-mo posttreatment follow-up; compared with usual community services	Improved youth functioning and school functioning, decreased substance use problems, and rearrests	Community therapists/ community provider	Standard
Sundell et al,[54] 2008	Swedish youth with conduct disorder (N = 156)	RCT; 7-mo postrecruitment; compared with usual child welfare services	No outcomes favoring either treatment condition; low treatment fidelity	Community therapists/ community provider: 4 sites	Standard
Glisson et al,[55] 2010	Juvenile offenders (N = 615)	RCT; 18-mo postrecruitment follow-up; compared with usual services	Decreased out-of-home placements	Community therapists/ community provider	Standard
Butler et al,[8] 2011	British juvenile offenders (N = 108)	RCT; 18-mo postrecruitment follow-up; compared with a tailored range of extensive and multicomponent evidence-based interventions	Reduced offenses and placements, self- and parent-reported delinquency, psychopathic symptoms; improved parenting	Community therapists/ community provider	Standard

Study	Population	Design	Outcomes	Therapists/Comparison	Model
Asscher et al,[7] 2013	Dutch youth with severe and violent antisocial behavior (N = 256)	RCT; 6 mo postrecruitment follow-up; compared with usual services	Decreased antisocial behavior; increased parental sense of competence, positive discipline, and relationship quality; increased youth association with positive peers	Community therapists/ community provider	Standard
Henggeler et al,[15] 2006	Substance abusing and dependent juvenile offenders in Drug Court (N = 161)	RCT; 12-mo postrecruitment follow-up; compared 4 conditions: Family Court with Usual Services, Drug Court with Usual Services, Drug Court with Standard MST, Drug Court with MST and CM	MST enhanced substance use outcomes for alcohol and marijuana	Community therapists/ university	MST-SA
Weiss et al,[56] 2013	Adolescents with serious conduct problems in self-contained classrooms (N = 164)	RCT; 18-mo and 2.5-y postrecruitment follow-up; compared with usual services	Reduced externalizing problems but not arrests; decreased school absences; improved parenting and parental mental health symptoms	Community therapists/ university	Standard
Henggeler et al,[9] 1999; Brown et al,[41] 1999; Henggeler et al,[42] 2002	Substance- abusing and dependent delinquents (N = 118)	RCT; 6-mo, 11-mo, and 4-y postrecruitment follow-up; compared with usual community services	At 6-mo postrecruitment: increased attendance in regular school settings At 11-mo postrecruitment: decreased drug use, out-of-home placement, criminal arrests (nonsignificant); treatment adherence was related to decreased drug use and other outcomes At 4-y follow-up: decreased violent crime; increased marijuana abstinence	Community therapists/ university	MST-SA

(continued on next page)

Table 1
(continued)

Study	Sample	Design	Findings	Provider/Setting	MST Type
Brunk et al,[43] 1987	Maltreating families (N = 33)	RCT; posttreatment evaluations; compared with behavioral parent training	Improved parent-child interactions	Graduate students/ university	MST-CAN
Swenson et al,[16] 2010	Maltreating families (N = 86)	RCT; 16-mo postrecruitment follow-up; compared with group-based parent training and enhanced outpatient treatment	Decreased symptoms for youth and caregiver; improved parenting behaviors and social support; decreased out-of-home placements	Community therapists/ community provider	MST-CAN
Schaeffer et al,[44] 2013	Co-occurring parental substance abuse and child maltreatment (N = 43)	Single-group pre-, post-, and quasiexperimental designs; posttreatment follow-up for single group design and 24-mo postreferral follow-up for quasiexperimental design; compared with comprehensive community treatment	Posttreatment: reduced substance abuse and depression among mothers; improved parenting; decreased anxiety among youth 24-mo postreferral follow-up: decreased maltreatment and time youth spent in out-of-home placement	Community therapists/ community provider	MST-BSF Adaptation

and high client satisfaction. These effects are lasting, as demonstrated by a 22-year follow-up study showing that youth who received MST during adolescence had fewer felony arrests (violent and nonviolent), days incarcerated, divorces, and paternity or child support suits in adulthood.[40]

Multisystemic Therapy for Substance Abuse

An early study found that MST was superior to usual community services on improvements in substance use, school attendance, and out-of-home placement.[9,41] The group receiving MST continued to show superior results in terms of marijuana abstinence and engagement in violent crime 4 years later.[42] In a more recent clinical trial, integrating CM (referred to as MST-SA) enhanced the effectiveness of standard MST in treating adolescent substance abuse.[15] Thus, there is substantial evidence that MST-SA is effective and superior to standard MST for substance abusing adolescents.

Multisystemic Therapy for Child Abuse and Neglect

There have been 15 years of research on MST-CAN, including 2 randomized clinical trials (RCTs). The first RCT randomized 43 families with indicated abuse or neglect to either standard MST or Behavioral Parent Training.[43] MST showed more favorable effects on family problems, parent-child relations, and key parenting behaviors than did group-based parent training. The second RCT randomized 86 families who had indicated physical abuse to either MST-CAN or Enhanced Outpatient Therapy (EOT), which consisted of a parenting group plus extra efforts to engage the family in treatment.[16] At 16 months after baseline, MST-CAN was more effective than EOT in reducing internalizing problems, out-of-home placements, and (for those who were placed) changes in placement. Caregivers also had greater improvements in (1) psychiatric distress; (2) parenting associated with maltreatment; (3) use of nonviolent discipline; and (4) social support compared with parents receiving EOT. Fewer MST-CAN youth experienced reabuse, but base rates were low, and the difference was not statistically significant. These trials established MST-CAN as an evidence-based intervention. A related model, MST-Building Stronger Families (MST-BSF), was developed for families experiencing physical abuse and neglect plus serious parental substance misuse. Preliminary findings with MST-BSF are promising,[44] and an RCT is currently underway.

SUMMARY

Given the multidetermined nature of adolescent externalizing behaviors, effective interventions must target risk factors at the individual, family, school, and community levels. MST was designed specifically for this purpose and has been shown through decades of research to be effective for serious clinical problems that put adolescents at risk for out-of-home placement, including juvenile offending, serious externalizing behaviors, substance abuse, and parental physical abuse and neglect. Furthermore, recent research has focused on mechanisms for effective transportability and implementation of MST to community settings. MST researchers have demonstrated the importance of high treatment fidelity and pioneered a quality assurance system that allows for replication of positive outcomes in community settings through ongoing supervision and support from MST experts. Despite these significant advances, only 5% of serious juvenile offenders receive an evidence-based treatment in the United States,[45] indicating that an ongoing challenge for the field is to develop strategies for expanding access to effective treatments for these high-risk populations.

REFERENCES

1. Henggeler SW, Schoenwald SK, Borduin CM, et al. Multisystemic therapy for anti-social behavior in children and adolescents. 2nd edition. New York: Guilford; 2009.
2. Loeber R, Burke JD, Pardini DA. Development and etiology of disruptive and delinquent behavior. Annu Rev Clin Psychol 2009;5:291–310.
3. Thornberry TP, Krohn MD, editors. Taking stock of delinquency: an overview of findings from contemporary longitudinal studies. New York: Kluwer/Plenum; 2003.
4. Bronfenbrenner U. The ecology of human development: experiments by design and nature. Cambridge (MA): Harvard University Press; 1979.
5. Haley J. Problem solving therapy. San Francisco (CA): Jossey-Bass; 1987.
6. Minuchin S. Families and family therapy. Cambridge (MA): Harvard University Press; 1974.
7. Asscher JJ, Dekovic M, Manders WA, et al. A randomized controlled trial of the effectiveness of multisystemic therapy in the Netherlands: post-treatment changes and moderator effects. J Exp Criminol 2013;9:169–87.
8. Butler S, Baruch G, Hickley N, et al. A randomized controlled trial of MST a statutory therapeutic intervention for young offenders. J Am Acad Child Adolesc Psychiatry 2011;12:1220–35.
9. Henggeler SW, Pickrel SG, Brondino MJ. Multisystemic treatment of substance abusing and dependent delinquents: outcomes, treatment fidelity, and transportability. Ment Health Serv Res 1999;1:171–84.
10. Tighe A, Pistrang N, Casdagli L, et al. Multisystemic therapy for young offenders: families' experiences of therapeutic processes and outcomes. J Fam Psychol 2012;26:187–97.
11. Henggeler SW, Melton GB, Brondino MJ, et al. Multisystemic therapy with violent and chronic juvenile offenders and their families: the role of treatment fidelity in successful dissemination. J Consult Clin Psychol 1997;65:821–33.
12. Huey SJ, Henggeler SW, Brondino MJ, et al. Mechanisms of change in multisystemic therapy: reducing delinquent behavior through therapist adherence and improved family and peer functioning. J Consult Clin Psychol 2000;68:451–67.
13. Schoenwald SK, Carter RE, Chapman JE, et al. Therapist adherence and organizational effects on change in youth behavior problems one year after multisystemic therapy. Adm Policy Ment Health 2008;35:379–94.
14. Schoenwald SK, Chapman JE, Sheidow AJ, et al. Long-term youth criminal outcomes in MST transport: the impact of therapist adherence and organizational climate and structure. J Clin Child Adolesc Psychol 2009;38:91–105.
15. Henggeler SW, Halliday-Boykins CA, Cunningham PB, et al. Juvenile drug court: enhancing outcomes by integrating evidence-based treatments. J Consult Clin Psychol 2006;74:42–54.
16. Swenson CC, Schaeffer CM, Henggeler SW, et al. Multisystemic therapy for child abuse and neglect: a randomized effectiveness trial. J Fam Psychol 2010;24:497–507.
17. Dishion TJ, Kavanagh K. Intervening in adolescent problem behavior: a family-centered approach. New York: Guilford; 2003.
18. Barnes GM, Reifman AS, Farrell MP, et al. The effects of parenting on the development of alcohol misuse: a six-wave latent growth model. J Marriage Fam 1994; 62:175–86.
19. Gorman-Smith D, Tolan PH, Loeber R, et al. Relation of family problems to patterns of delinquent involvement among urban youth. J Abnorm Child Psychol 1998;26:319–33.

20. Steinberg L, Fletcher A, Darling N. Parental monitoring and peer influences on adolescent substance abuse. Pediatrics 1994;93:1060–4.
21. Farrell AD, Danish SJ. Peer drug associations and emotional restraint: causes or consequences of adolescents' drug use? J Consult Clin Psychol 1993;61:327–34.
22. Newcomb MD, Bentler PM. Substance use and abuse among children and teenagers. Am Psychol 1989;44:242–8.
23. Cyr C, Euser EM, Bakermans-Kranenburg MJ, et al. Attachment security and disorganization in maltreating and high-risk families: a series of meta-analyses. Dev Psychopathol 2010;22:87–108.
24. Hussey JM, Chang JJ, Kotch JB. Child maltreatment in the United States: prevalence, risk factors, and adolescent health consequences. Pediatrics 2006;118: 933–42.
25. Kim J, Cicchetti D, Rogosch FA, et al. Child maltreatment and trajectories of personality and behavioral functioning: implications for the development of personality disorder. Dev Psychopathol 2009;21:889–912.
26. Kolko DJ, Swenson CC. Assessing and treating physically abused children and their families: a cognitive-behavioral approach. Thousand Oaks (CA): Sage; 2002.
27. Sidebotham P, Heron J. Child maltreatment in the children of the nineties: a cohort study of risk factors. Child Abuse Negl 2006;30:497–522.
28. Appel AE, Holden GW. The occurrence of spouse and physical child abuse: a review and appraisal. J Fam Psychol 1998;12:578–99.
29. Black DA, Heyman RE, Slep AM. Risk factors for child physical abuse. Aggress Violent Behav 2001;6:121–88.
30. Crouch JL, Milner JS, Thomsen C. Childhood physical abuse, early social support, and risk for maltreatment: current social support as a mediator of risk for child physical abuse. Child Abuse Negl 2001;25:93–107.
31. Hebert S, Bor W, Swenson CC, et al. Improving collaboration: a qualitative assessment of inter-agency collaboration between a pilot Multisystemic Therapy Child Abuse and Neglect (MST-CAN) program and a child protection team. Australas Psychiatry 2014;22:370–3.
32. Lipovsky JA, Swenson CC, Ralston ME, et al. The abuse clarification process in the treatment of intrafamilial child abuse. Child Abuse Negl 1998;22:729–41.
33. Feindler EL. Adolescent anger control: review and critique. Prog Behav Modif 1990;26:11–59.
34. Robin AL, Bedway M, Gilroy M. Problem solving communication training. In: LeCroy CW, editor. Handbook of child and adolescent treatment manuals. New York: Lexington Books; 1994. p. 92–125.
35. Foa EB, Rothbaum BO. Treating the trauma of rape: cognitive behavioral therapy for PTSD. New York: Guilford; 1998.
36. Tuten M, Jones HE, Schaeffer CM, et al. Reinforcement-based treatment (RBT): a practical guide for the behavioral treatment of drug addiction. Washington, DC: American Psychological Association; 2012.
37. Swenson CC, Schaeffer CM. Multisystemic Therapy for Child Abuse and Neglect. In: Rubin A, editor. Clinician's guide to evidence-based practice: programs and interventions for maltreated children and families at risk. Hoboken (NJ): John Wiley & Sons; 2012. p. 31–41.
38. Blueprints. Blueprints database standards. University of Colorado, Center for the Study and Prevention of Violence. Boulder (CO): Blueprints; 2013.
39. MST Services. Multisystemic Therapy (MST) research at a glance: published MST outcome, implementation, and benchmarking studies. 2014. Available at: http://www.mstservices.com/proven-results/proven-results. Accessed October 12, 2014.

40. Sawyer AM, Borduin CM. Effects of MST through midlife: a 21.9-year follow-up to a randomized clinical trial with serious and violent juvenile offenders. J Consult Clin Psychol 2011;79:643–52.

41. Brown TL, Henggeler SW, Schoenwald SK, et al. Multisystemic treatment of substance abusing and dependent juvenile delinquents: effects on school attendance at posttreatment and 6-month follow-up. Child Serv Soc Pol Res Pract 1999;2:81–93.

42. Henggeler SW, Clingempeel WG, Brondino MJ, et al. Four-year follow-up of multisystemic therapy with substance abusing and dependent juvenile offenders. J Am Acad Child Adolesc Psychiatry 2002;41:868–74.

43. Brunk M, Henggeler SW, Whelan JP. A comparison of multisystemic therapy and parent training in the brief treatment of child abuse and neglect. J Consult Clin Psychol 1987;55:311–8.

44. Schaeffer CM, Swenson CC, Tuerk EH, et al. Comprehensive treatment for co-occurring child maltreatment and parental substance abuse: outcomes from a 24-month pilot study of the MST-Building Stronger Families program. Child Abuse Negl 2013;37:596–607.

45. Henggeler SW, Schoenwald SK. Evidence based interventions for juvenile offenders and juvenile justice policies that support them. Soc Policy Rep 2011;25:3–25.

46. Henggeler SW, Rodick JD, Borduin CM, et al. Multisystemic treatment of juvenile offenders: effects on adolescent behavior and family interactions. Dev Psychol 1986;22:132–41.

47. Henggeler SW, Melton GB, Smith LA. Family preservation using multisystemic therapy: an effective alternative to incarcerating serious juvenile offenders. J Consult Clin Psychol 1992;60:953–61.

48. Henggeler SW, Melton GB, Smith LA, et al. Family preservation using multisystemic treatment: long-term follow-up to a clinical trial with serious juvenile offenders. J Child Fam Stud 1993;2:283–93.

49. Borduin CM, Mann BJ, Cone LT, et al. Multisystemic treatment of serious juvenile offenders: long-term prevention of criminality and violence. J Consult Clin Psychol 1995;63:569–78.

50. Schaeffer CM, Borduin CM. Long-term follow-up to a randomized clinical trial of multisystemic therapy with serious and violent juvenile offenders. J Consult Clin Psychol 2005;73:445–53.

51. Ogden T, Halliday-Boykins CA. Multisystemic treatment of antisocial adolescents in Norway: replication of clinical outcomes outside of the US. Child Adolesc Ment Health 2004;9:77–83.

52. Ogden T, Hagen KA. Multisystemic therapy of serious behaviour problems in youth: sustainability of therapy effectiveness two years after intake. J Child Adolesc Ment Health 2006;11:142–9.

53. Timmons-Mitchell J, Bender MB, Kishna MA, et al. An independent effectiveness trial of multisystemic therapy with juvenile justice youth. J Clin Child Adolesc Psychol 2006;35:227–36.

54. Sundell K, Hansson K, Lofholm CE, et al. The transportability of multisystemic therapy to Sweden: short-term results from a randomized trial of conduct-disordered youths. J Fam Psychol 2008;22:550–6.

55. Glisson C, Schoenwald SK, Hemmelgarn A, et al. Randomized trial of MST and ARC in a two-level EBT implementation strategy. J Consult Clin Psychol 2010; 78:537–50.

56. Weiss B, Han S, Harris V, et al. An independent randomized clinical trial of multisystemic therapy with non-court-referred adolescents with serious conduct problems. J Consult Clin Psychol 2013;81:1027–39.

Family-based Treatment of Child and Adolescent Eating Disorders

Sarah Forsberg, PsyD*, James Lock, MD, PhD

KEYWORDS

- Eating disorders • Anorexia nervosa • Bulimia nervosa • Family-based treatment

KEY POINTS

- Twelve-month prevalence rates of eating disorders (EDs) among adolescents are as high as 2.6% in bulimia nervosa (BN) and 1% in anorexia nervosa (AN), with subthreshold presentations occurring at much higher rates.
- AN has the highest mortality of any psychiatric disorder and all EDs are punctuated by social impairment (loss of role functioning), psychiatric comorbidity, with high rates of suicide.
- Family treatment models, specifically family-based treatment (FBT) is the best evidence-based approach for adolescents with AN.
- FBT is a parental-empowerment model that supports parents in disrupting the harmful behaviors that maintain the ED.
- Preliminary data from systematic research support the use of FBT in the treatment of adolescent BN.

Eating disorders (EDs) have long been treated in a family context and inclusion of family members in therapeutic interventions of these adolescents is considered best practice.[1,2] This recommendation highlights an important paradigm shift away from the early view that parents were the worst possible attendants in caring for their child with anorexia nervosa (AN), because they are now considered a central resource in bringing about recovery.[3] As early as the 1970s, many family therapists took interest in the family dynamics that were thought to maintain the presence of AN. For example,

Disclosures: J. Lock: Training Institute for Child and Adolescent Eating Disorders (codirector), Guilford Press (royalties), Oxford Press (royalties), Optum Health (scientific advisory board), Global Foundation for Eating Disorders (grant support), NEDA (scientific advisory board), Davis Foundation (grant support), NIH grants (R01 MH079978-01A2, R34 MH093493, R21 MH096779-01, R34 MH101281, R03 MH096144-01A1), Centers for Discovery (scientific advisory board), Recovery Record (unpaid consultant), Sedgwick LLP (expert testimony).
Department of Psychiatry and Behavioral Sciences, Stanford University, 401 Quarry Road, Stanford, CA 94305, USA
* Corresponding author.
E-mail address: sforsberg@stanford.edu

Child Adolesc Psychiatric Clin N Am 24 (2015) 617–629
http://dx.doi.org/10.1016/j.chc.2015.02.012
1056-4993/15/$ – see front matter © 2015 Elsevier Inc. All rights reserved.

childpsych.theclinics.com

Abbreviations	
AN	Anorexia nervosa
BN	Bulimia nervosa
CBT-GSH	Guided self-help version of cognitive behavior therapy
ED	Eating disorder
EE	Expressed emotion
FBT	Family-based treatment
FBT-BN	FBT manualized for bulimia nervosa
SPT	Supportive psychotherapy
SyFT	Family systems therapy

Salvador Minuchin, the founder of structural family therapy, viewed the manifestation of AN as a means of supporting the maintenance of pathologic processes characterizing so-called psychosomatic families. Familial patterns of overprotectiveness, rigidity, enmeshment, and conflict avoidance were putatively addressed in part by restoring intergenerational boundaries and establishing effective conflict management.[4] Minuchin and colleagues[4] were the first to publish findings suggesting that family therapy could be helpful for adolescent AN, and their report of success with most of their patients generated interest in further exploration.

An alternative view of family treatment of adolescent AN was based in the Milan school of systemic family therapy developed around the same time by Selvini Palazzoli.[5] The therapeutic stance in systemic family therapy is nondirective and promotes family exploration and autonomy in identifying changes. This approach is thought to circumvent family resistance to outside interventions, allowing the therapist to join the family in a supportive role. Other schools of family therapy also contributed to the development of a specific family therapy model for adolescent AN, including strategic family therapy[6] and narrative family therapy.[7,8]

These early family models provided the groundwork for the development of what is now called family-based treatment (FBT). The approach was developed at the Institute of Psychiatry and integrated structural, systemic, strategic, and narrative family therapy elements that were thought to be practical in their application to AN.[9] Although early models of family therapy are a far cry from the pathologic view of families that encouraged so-called parentectomy, both structural and strategic theory insinuate causality, even though this is not directly communicated. In contrast, a central tenet explicitly stated in FBT is that families are not to blame for their child's AN, and are instead considered the most helpful and positive resource in bringing about recovery. Thus, the therapist works to shift the family's focus away from causal mechanisms of AN, and must externalize and maintain an agnostic perspective throughout treatment themselves.

FBT[10,11] is a manualized treatment. At its core, FBT empowers parents to directly manage ED behaviors (eg, excessive exercise, dietary restriction, purging, and binge eating) that maintain AN. This treatment includes positioning parents as authorities on their child, with the therapist serving as consultant around the nuances of AN. Family structures are only modified if they interfere with parental ability to support their child in gaining weight.

The application of FBT has predominantly focused on individuals with AN; however, given the significant overlap in symptoms across ED diagnoses, more recent efforts have examined its utility in treating adolescent bulimia nervosa (BN). Although individuals with BN tend to present to treatment at a later average age than their AN counterparts, they too are typically nested in the family.[12] FBT manualized for BN (FBT-BN) largely draws on the theory outlined for AN. Thus, parents are encouraged to use strategies that arrest binge eating and purging behaviors. BN is more ego dystonic and distressing to the adolescent, whereas AN is often experienced as consistent with the person's identity, therein challenging healthy decision making and requiring significant parental control. The difference in presentation of BN thus necessitates a collaborative process between the parent-adolescent dyad. These modifications are outlined in detail in a manual published by Le Grange and Lock[13] and are further elaborated later.

EMPIRICAL FINDINGS ON FAMILY-BASED TREATMENT OF EATING DISORDERS
Family-based Treatment of Anorexia Nervosa

Despite the long-standing tradition of studying family process and treatment of EDs, the empirical support for this practice is sparse. However, most empirical studies of adolescent AN have included variants of FBT in its current iteration, and, in light of this work, clinical guidelines recommend family treatment as a front-line approach.[1,14]

There are 7 published randomized controlled studies of adolescent AN, all of which have included FBT. Compared with individual modalities, FBT shows better clinical outcomes, maintained across follow-up points.[9,15–17] Data suggest that family therapy may confer a specific benefit to those with a shorter duration of illness (<3 years) and an onset before age 18 years.[9,15] Individuals receiving FBT were less likely to need hospitalization and had lower rates of relapse at 1-year follow-up.[16,18] In the largest trial to date, FBT was compared with family systems therapy (SyFT). Both groups achieved similar rates of remission in ED symptoms, but FBT promoted more rapid weight gain, required less hospital use, and was more cost-effective than SyFT.[19] These preliminary findings provide strong support for continued exploration of family therapy with this group, and also suggest areas for enhancement or adaptation to serve those who do not respond.

Additional randomized controlled trials, open trials, and case series reveal important information about adaptations to FBT, dose, and special populations. FBT for adolescent AN has been shown to be effective when delivered in a shorter dose (10-session format delivered over 6 months vs 20 sessions delivered over 12 months); however, individuals from nonintact families, and those who are more obsessional about food and weight benefited from the longer format.[20] In cases of families with significant parental criticism directed at the adolescent (high levels of expressed emotion [EE]), seeing parents separately from their child promoted improved outcomes.[18] However, recent data suggest that families with high EE can also be treated effectively in traditional, conjoint FBT.[21,22] Further, FBT seems to be more successful in treating those individuals with higher eating-related psychopathology with obsessive-compulsive features, than individual treatment.[23] Individuals with comorbid psychiatric illness also show lower rates of remission and dropout in FBT.[24] Although younger age is a predictor of good outcome, age has not been found to moderate treatment outcome in existing trials, and results of a case series show similar positive effects of FBT for children aged 12 years and younger.[25]

Family-based Treatment of Bulimia Nervosa

The empirical examination of the treatment of adolescent BN has been severely neglected. Only 2 randomized trials have been conducted to date, both including a form of family therapy. The first used a model of family therapy loosely based on FBT, in which families included any close other in the adolescent's life. There were no significant differences detected between those receiving family treatment compared with those in a guided self-help version of cognitive behavior therapy (CBT-GSH).[26] Primary outcome in BN studies is defined by abstinence from binge/purge behaviors, and rates were comparable across treatment arms. The other trial compared FBT-BN with individual supportive psychotherapy (SPT). At end of treatment, subjects receiving FBT-BN had similar abstinence rates to those receiving family treatment in the Schmidt and colleagues[26] study and FBT was statistically superior to SPT. Further, FBT brought about greater improvement in all measures of core ED symptoms.[27] Follow-up studies designed to differentiate response to FBT among patient subgroups have collected preliminary data (Table 1).

IMPLEMENTATION OF FAMILY-BASED TREATMENT OF EATING DISORDERS
Family-based Treatment of Anorexia Nervosa

A set of fundamental assumptions underlies all therapeutic interventions within FBT (Table 2). In summary, FBT posits that there is no known cause of AN. Therapists recognize that the cause of AN may exist somewhere in the intersection of a multitude of biological, social, and psychological factors with unknown relative influence. Most importantly, families are not to blame for the emergence of the disorder and the therapists must remain agnostic while helping the family to do the same. Second, AN is not under the control of the adolescent. As in disease models of mental illness, AN is treated initially as a medical condition with emphasis on addressing the serious medical consequences of the disorder. Parents are thus placed in charge of providing their child with medicine in the form of food in order to restore healthy organ functioning and cognition. This regressed and medically fragile state is seen as limited and, as health is restored, greater adolescent autonomy is negotiated as developmentally appropriate. Thus, conditions of the illness require externalization; as the family is supported in viewing the ED behaviors and emotional and social consequences of AN as endogenous to the disease, they are better equipped to separate the illness from their child. In this way, they may take control over the ED behaviors while supporting and reinforcing all signs of healthy development.

Adaptations for Bulimia Nervosa

Parental empowerment is thought to be critical to change in FBT for BN as in treatment of AN. Despite similarities between these disorders, unique features of BN inform modifications to the model. Individuals with AN and BN are preoccupied with shape and weight to the extent that these become a primary focus of self-evaluation and drive compensatory behaviors. In AN, there is a significant discrepancy between reality (severe emaciation) and perception, whereas in BN this contrast is not as striking. These differences may in part explain the tendency for BN to feel dystonic to an individual's sense of self, and thus highly distressing. In general, adolescents with BN experience significant guilt and shame around bingeing and purging behaviors, and the lack of success in controlling their weight through dieting. These emotions often precipitate increased withdrawal from friends and family, thus strengthening the illness in its isolation. Similar to AN, although typically to a lesser degree, individuals with BN may minimize the seriousness of their illness, further impairing their ability to manage symptoms independently of parental support. As in FBT-AN, therapists are in a consultative role, providing significant psychoeducation with the aim of absolving the adolescents of responsibility for their actions, and alleviating family guilt and shame. The primary difference is the extent to which the adolescent is invited to join parents in collaborating around efforts to disrupt binge eating, purging, and irregular eating patterns. Adolescents with BN are typically viewed as more on track developmentally, with a greater degree of insight. Their

Table 1
Outpatient psychotherapy trials of family treatments for adolescent AN and BN

Trial	Treatment Type	N	Mean Age (y)	Outcome
Adolescent AN				
Russell et al,[9] 1987	Family therapy vs supportive individual therapy	21	15.3	[a]Family therapy, 90%[b] Individual, 18%
Le Grange et al,[18] 1992	Whole family vs separated family therapy	18	15.3	[a]68% overall; no differences between groups
Robin et al,[28] 1999	Family therapy vs individual therapy	37	13.9	[a]Family therapy, 81%[b] Individual therapy, 66%
Eisler et al,[29] 2000	Whole family vs separated family therapy	40	15.5	[a]63% overall; no differences between groups
Lock et al,[20] 2005; Lock et al,[30] 2006	Family treatment (FBT), 6-mo vs 12-mo dose	86	15.1	[a]96% overall; no difference in weight change or psychological change between groups at end of treatment or 4-y follow-up
Lock et al,[16] 2010	Family therapy (FBT) vs individual therapy (AFT)	121	14.4	[a]FBT, 89%[b] AFT, 67% [c]Full remission EOT: FBT, 40% AFT, 19% 1-y follow-up: FBT, 50%[b] AFT, 20%
Agras et al,[19] early view	FBT vs family systems (SyFT)	164		[c]EOT: FBT, 33.1% SyFT, 25.3% [c]1-y follow-up: FBT, 40.7% SyFT, 39%
Adolescent BN				
Schmidt et al,[26] 2007	Family therapy vs CBT-GSH	85	17.9	[d]Family, 26% CBT-GSH, 42%
Le Grange et al,[27] 2007	FBT vs supportive individual therapy	80	16.1	[d]FBT, 40% Individual, 19%

Abbreviation: EOT, end of treatment.
[a] Outcome defined as rates of individuals meeting Morgan-Russell good/intermediate threshold (>85% of expected body weight in AN).
[b] $P<.05$.
[c] Full remission means greater than or equal to 95% of expected body weight.
[d] Abstinence rates from binge/purge behaviors.
Adapted from Lock J, Le Grange D. Treatment manual for anorexia nervosa, second edition: a family based approach. New York: The Guilford Press; 2013; with permission.

Table 2
Principles of FBT for EDs

Principle	Goal	Related Interventions	Modifications for FBT-BN
Agnosticism	Decrease parental guilt; decrease blame Facilitate focus on current maintaining features of the ED	Highlight lack of causal data and dispel myths Emphasize evidence of successful outcome through disruption of symptoms rather than insight on cause	None
Symptom focus	Disrupt behaviors that maintain ED	Review weight progress/binge/purge frequency at outset of session Use data as guide for detailed discussion of successes and challenges in progress	Focus on normalizing eating patterns and decreasing binge/purge behaviors rather than weight restoration because individuals with BN are typically at normal weights
Consultative therapeutic stance	Increase parental alignment Increase parental self-efficacy	Encourage parents to work through solutions to current challenges Provide input as gathered through expertise on EDs (garnered through work with parents and research base) Assist family in understanding nutritional needs of their child	Adolescent may be more involved in problem-solving process as input is consistent with recovery-based goals
Parental empowerment	Reposition parents as authority on their child Increase parental self-efficacy	Place parents in charge of disrupting ED symptoms/meal management Reinforce positive steps taken to disrupt ED Frame challenges as opportunities to problem solve and adapt skill set	Adolescent may participate as appropriate in decisions about how to work on goals
Externalization of illness	Separate the illness from the patient Decrease familial criticism Align with intact healthy part of the adolescent	Use of Venn diagram to represent healthy characteristics/behaviors of the adolescent, ED-related characteristics and behaviors, and their overlap Encourage adolescent to consider both positive and negative impacts of the ED	Adolescent with BN may more easily separate the illness from their own sense of self (eg, are more likely to view BN as egodystonic)

increased independence is acknowledged within the treatment; if regressed, maladaptive decisions regarding food and eating are highlighted as areas for increased parental intervention.

Structure of Treatment

FBT for AN typically takes place over the course of 10 to 20 sessions spaced over 6 to 12 months. As noted, shorter forms of FBT can be just as effective, and recent data suggest that weight gain (around 2–2.5 kg [4–5 pounds]) is the strongest identified predictor of recovery.[31,32] Therefore, weight restoration in the home environment is a primary aim, and it is determined by evaluation of various data points (historical growth curves, normative growth curves, resumption of hormonal function and menses among girls).

For FBT-BN a typical course of treatment is 20 sessions over 6 months,[13] with most time spent in phase I focusing on resumption of healthy eating patterns and decreased binge/purge behaviors. Success is determined by the therapist's ability to align parents in actively disrupting ED symptoms. The negotiation of parental involvement varies from family to family but often includes parental encouragement and provision of 3 meals and 2 to 3 snacks each day, parental monitoring and engagement in distraction after mealtimes, and temporary removal of binge foods from the home. Each session begins with a 10-minute to 15-minute meeting with the adolescent to obtain weight, assess frequency of binge/purge behaviors, and establish agenda items. Weight and binge/purge frequency are tracked on logs and shared with the family as markers of progress and challenge. Discrepancies between parent and adolescent reports of these behaviors are addressed as the log is shared when the family session convenes. In engaging the family in management of ED symptoms, the therapist is cautious in balancing efforts to align parents in a position of authority, while facilitating developmentally appropriate input from the adolescent. Recall that in treatment of AN the therapist is clear that they will not engage with the adolescent in negotiations about weight gain, a distinct difference between the two models.

Treatment Overview and Case Example

The following case example highlights key interventions and modifications to address challenges common to work with this population.

PRESENTING INFORMATION

Alexa is a Mexican-American 15-year-old with a 2-year history of AN punctuated by severe dietary restriction, occasional objective binges, ongoing self-induced vomiting, and excessive exercise. She had 2 previous hospitalizations for bradycardia and orthostasis, and was referred directly from an inpatient medical unit to the outpatient program. Her weight was below the 10th percentile for age and height; and she had a 1.5-year history of amenorrhea. The family of origin included her mother, grandmother, and 4-year-old brother.

Phase I Key Interventions

In the first session the therapist strives to accomplish the following tasks:
- Gather family history related to the impact of AN on the family
- Obtain history of the development of AN
- Orchestrate an intense scene surrounding the severe physical, social, and emotional consequences of AN to mobilize the parents
- Reduce parental guilt and blame
- Charge parents with the task of weight restoration of their child

- Externalize the illness
- Modify parental/sibling criticism
- Remain agnostic

Session 2: the family meal.

- Take a history of family meal preparation, serving, discussion
- Assist the family in understanding the nutritional needs of their child
- Align parents in their efforts to refeed
- Encourage the parents to assist their child in taking 1 more bite
- Keep the focus on AN and eating behaviors
- Align siblings in supportive role

The remainder of phase I continually incorporates the focus on parental empowerment, agnosticism, and externalization. In addition, the therapist:

- Provides ongoing feedback on weight and uses weight to guide in-session targets
- Directs therapeutic discussion toward food, eating, and their management
- Supports parental efforts at weight restoration

PHASE I CHALLENGES

From the first family meeting, it became clear to the therapist that Alexa's mother was experiencing guilt for being less available to Alexa after having returned to night school in addition to having a full-time job. In contrast, when Alexa refused to eat by leaving the table, screaming, crying, or threatening to run away, her mother quickly became critical, openly sharing her belief that her daughter was manipulating her in order to get attention. Thus, the therapist made significant efforts at the outset of treatment to redirect criticism toward the illness in its persistent grip over Alexa. He did this through assisting the family in creating a Venn diagram to illustrate the extent to which Alexa, who the family identified as empathic, an advocate for others, hard working, and a talented artist, had become overcome by AN (which they eventually called The Squid). This useful metaphor allowed the therapist to redirect family criticism quickly and refocus attention on developing strategies to disrupt behaviors that were maintaining AN (eg, endless bargaining about nutritional needs or family acquiescence in response to threats that she would throw up anyway after a meal). Given the family structure (single, working parent), and their limited financial resources, the therapist problem solved with the family to creatively identify sources of support. Alexa's mother was able to work with her school to take a leave of absence. Her grandmother was comfortable in the role of providing meals and readily increased the caloric density, often being the first to provide suggestions for meals. During meals, Alexa's mother and grandmother worked together, taking turns sitting with her in the midst of emotional outbursts, which required a firm, quiet, and patient presence. The family was able to practice responding to these challenges during the family meal session, whereby the therapist encouraged them to practice their own self-care to maintain the emotional resources required to consistently return their focus to refeeding once Alexa's distress had subsided. The mother and grandmother discovered and used their own language as a reminder to stay focused, persistent, and to express empathy, and would remind Alexa that, "We know how hard this is for you, and we cannot let The Squid tighten his grip; we will sit with you until you finish your meal." Further, the family realized that meals at relatives' homes were much easier, because Alexa was more compliant, and often more relaxed. The family scheduled meals outside of the home, and began to invite relatives and a neighbor to the home as Alexa became more comfortable.

Phase II Key Interventions

As the patient with AN begins to eat with more ease, allowing parental refeeding efforts without conflict, the family and therapist discuss readiness for phase II. Phase II generally does not begin until there has been sufficient weight progress (typically gaining to within 90%–95% of expected body weight).

Key interventions:

- Shape developmentally appropriate independence around eating, which might include the adolescent:
  ○ Selecting a part of the meal
  ○ Choosing between 2 equivalent snacks
  ○ Portioning with parental oversight
  ○ Eating a meal with a friend
  ○ Eating at school without parental supervision
  ○ Introducing some physical activity

Phase III Key Interventions

Readiness for phase III is determined based on attainment and stabilization of a healthy weight, as well as behavioral progress in resumption of independence around eating. Here the therapist assists the family in:

- Shifting the focus to developmental challenges and family concerns, which may include:
  ○ Dating
  ○ Schoolwork and time management
  ○ Peer relationships
  ○ Family conflict resolution and problem solving
  ○ Other concerning behaviors or comorbid psychiatric symptoms
- Encouraging family generalization of skills toward other non-ED challenges
- Reviewing a relapse prevention plan

CHALLENGES AND OUTCOME

Once the family learned that they could tolerate, and wait out AN outbursts, and modified the environment (requiring Alexa leave the bathroom door cracked after meals, requiring she sit with her grandmother or mother, having a family member sit next to her during mealtimes), AN slowly loosened its grip. The decrease in family criticism and strength in empathizing with Alexa's struggle allowed greater connection in moments when Alexa sought their support (which gradually occurred more frequently following difficult meals). The family began to engage in activities (going for short walks, playing board games, watching their favorite comedy) that allowed connection and a means of practicing emotion regulation following distressing meals. The therapist helped the family anticipate challenges that AN might present as they intensified their efforts, thus the family was not as surprised when they found that Alexa had been hiding food, and were able to frame this as being external to Alexa's control. Alexa responded well to rewards and looked forward to spending more time on her own with friends. Thus, early checks on independence included attending movies with friends and eating lunch on her own at school, instead of with a school nurse. When her weight decreased following introduction of minimal independence, the family regrouped and brainstormed strategies to support healthy independence without encouraging AN (asking a school counselor to check in with Alexa throughout lunch). In Alexa's case, the motivation to be on her own was often sufficient to overcome initial setbacks. As she gradually returned to full physical activity (first partial participation in physical education, the addition of brief walks with her mother, and eventually return to tennis practice) she began to struggle as her body required additional nutrition. Thus, the family increased supervision of an extra evening snack, as opposed to decreasing physical activity. Although Alexa expressed anger around having to again increase her intake, she preferred this to not being able to play tennis.

Toward the end of treatment, the family reflected on ongoing struggles (setting limits with regard to curfew, use of social media, and negative sibling interactions). The therapist provided education about typical adolescent development and normalized Alexa's increasing attempts at negotiation and pushing limits. The mother often saw Alexa's increased argumentativeness as a direct attack on her, and in finding Alexa had lied to her on a few occasions, took this to mean her daughter did not respect her. Further, Alexa often took her mother's anger at her to mean she had failed more globally, leaving little space for acquisition of new skills. The therapist encouraged the family to engage in conversation rather than reverting to giving in or coming down too hard. The family found education about adolescent development informative, and over time their communication became less reactive and more exploratory, leaving room for negotiation and increasing autonomy. Further, the family worked to separate their fears about relapse from typical parental apprehension and concern about increasing independence. By the end of treatment (9 months, 22 sessions), Alexa had resumed a normal menstrual cycle, and was maintaining a weight that was on track with historical weight trajectories (40th body mass index percentile). Her ED cognitions emerged when exposed to foods she had first eliminated (sweets), as she expressed fear of bingeing, although since she began eating regularly she had not experienced objective binge episodes. Thus, toward the end of treatment, her family worked to gradually introduce these foods with greater oversight initially. Alexa was able to build mastery in eating these without feeling she lost control after regular exposures. By the end of treatment, although she struggled with occasional anxiety related to changes in her body, her interest and investment in peer relationships, exploring dating, playing tennis, and staying in school, coupled with strengthened family relationships and communication, were positive buffers against relapse.

Common Challenges

There are many common dilemmas therapists face in conducting FBT. Often, families and therapists alike become concerned about and/or distracted by the presence of comorbidity. In these instances, it is imperative for all parties to consider the extent to which symptoms of anxiety or depression, for example, are correlates of dysregulated or restrictive eating and their effects on energy, mood, and sleep. Therapists must provide a strong rationale to families for maintaining their focus on ED symptoms, with attention paid to comorbidity inasmuch as it interferes with restoration of health. Should threats to safety arise (eg, suicidal ideation or self-injury), the therapist will need to prioritize these concerns over eating disorder behaviors until they are resolved. In RCTs to date, AN patients with greater comorbidity were more likely to drop out of treatment (however to a lesser extent in FBT than individual treatment), and those with greater symptom severity (eating-related obsessions and compulsions) benefited from a longer course of treatment.[21,30,33] However, even with significant rates of comorbidity seen in these RCTs, secondary diagnoses do not appear to differentially impact (moderate) treatment outcome.[34]

Family differences (constitution, organization, and symptomology) warrant attention in FBT. An individual approach on occasion may be preferred in the context of high family criticism directed at the adolescent, as it has been shown to predict dropout in FBT.[33] When criticism toward the adolescent arises, the therapist prioritizes defusing, reshaping, and encouraging family use of externalization to reduce blame. In cases where a family presents a high level of expressed emotion (EE) in the form of criticism, separated FBT can be as effective as conjoint treatment.[35] Nonintact families are capable of meeting the demands of management of food and eating; however, therapists must often work harder to ensure these families have access to support. In the case of single-parent families, the therapist may engage more actively in the problem-solving and decision-making process, and often encourages parents to identify alternative supports (school nurses or counsellors, close friends, and other family members).

Evaluation of Outcome

Outcome in FBT for AN and BN is measured by examining eating disorder behavior, weight progress, and resumption of healthy physical function through medical examination. In AN, the primary goal is full weight restoration and a return to premorbid growth and development. Full remission is defined as attaining a weight that is 95% of expected body weight for age and height.[36] It is also often important to consider previous growth patterns prior to development of the ED, as in some cases individuals may have tracked above or below the 50th percentile for weight. Early weight gain (approximately 4–5 pounds within the first month of treatment) is a good prognostic indicator of full recovery at the end of treatment for adolescents with AN. In BN, abstinence from binge/purge behavior is the primary indicator of full remission. In both groups, being able to maintain healthy eating patterns with parental oversight that is more developmentally typical is an indicator of a good outcome. In FBT, psychological recovery (absence of ED cognitions) is also a goal; however, it is not uncommon for these symptoms to persist beyond weight restoration, typically normalizing around 1-year later.[17]

Currently, adaptations to the standard dose of treatment are under consideration for adolescent AN for application with those individuals who do not make weight progress early in treatment. A recent observational study suggests that certain family behavior during the family meal session may help to identify those who may be challenged to progress and thus require adaptations or alternative treatments.[37] However, at this juncture, there are few convincing data to accurately predict who is likely to benefit from FBT; thus, therapists must use good clinical judgment, evaluating patient safety, symptom severity, and parental capacity in determining when to pursue alternative treatment models.

SUMMARY

FBT is the best evidence-based treatment of adolescents with short-duration AN. Although additional studies are needed to refine the understanding of FBT, improve response rates to FBT, and identify alternative treatment to FBT, therapists working with this age group should be familiar with this approach. In the case of adolescent AN, parental involvement in the weight restoration process with early weight gain seems to be critical, and shows improved rates of recovery compared with an individual approach designed to promote adolescent autonomy. In BN, support of FBT is more limited, but the approach seems feasible, acceptable, and effective.

REFERENCES

1. National Institute for Clinical Excellence. Core interventions in the treatment and management of anorexia nervosa, bulimia nervosa, and binge eating disorder. London: British Psychological Society; 2004.
2. American Psychiatric Association. Practice guideline for the treatment of patients with eating disorders: third edition: American Psychiatric Association. Am J Psychiatry 2006;163:4–54.
3. Gull W. Anorexia nervosa (apepsia hysteria, anorexia hysteria). Transactions of the Clinical Society of London 1874;7:22–8.
4. Minuchin S, Rosman B, Baker I. Psychosomatic families: anorexia nervosa in context. Cambridge (MA): Harvard University Press; 1978.
5. Selvini Palazzoli M. Self-starvation: from the intrapsychic to the transpersonal approach. London: Chaucer; 1974.
6. Haley J. Uncommon therapy: the psychiatric techniques of Milton H. Erickson. New York: Norton; 1973.
7. White M, Epston D. Narrative means to therapeutic ends. New York: WW Norton; 1990.

8. White M. Anorexia nervosa: a cybernetic perspective. Fam Ther Collect 1987;20: 117–29.
9. Russell G, Szmukler G, Dare C, et al. An evaluation of family therapy in anorexia nervosa and bulimia nervosa. Arch Gen Psychiatry 1987;44(12):1047–56.
10. Lock J, Le Grange D. Treatment manual for anorexia nervosa: a family-based approach. 2nd edition. New York: Guilford Press; 2012.
11. Lock J, Le Grange D, Agras WS, et al. Treatment manual for anorexia nervosa: a family-based approach. New York: Guilford Press; 2001.
12. Swanson S, Crow S, Le Grange D, et al. Prevalence and correlates of eating disorders in adolescents. Results from the national comorbidity survey replication adolescent supplement. Arch Gen Psychiatry 2011;68:714–23.
13. Le Grange D, Lock J. Treating bulimia in adolescence: a family-based approach. New York: Guilford Press; 2007.
14. Le Grange D, Lock J, Loeb K, et al. Academy for eating disorders position paper: the role of the family in eating disorders. Int J Eat Disord 2010;43(1):1–5.
15. Eisler I, Dare C, Russell GF, et al. Family and individual therapy in anorexia nervosa: a 5-year follow-up. Arch Gen Psychiatry 1997;54(11):1025–30.
16. Lock J, Le Grange D, Agras W, et al. Randomized clinical trial comparing family-based treatment with adolescent-focused individual therapy for adolescents with anorexia nervosa. Arch Gen Psychiatry 2010;67(10):1025–32.
17. Le Grange D, Lock J, Accurso E, et al. Relapse from remission at two-to-four-year follow-up in two treatments for adolescent anorexia nervosa. J Am Acad Child Adolesc Psychiatry 2014;53(11):1162–7.
18. Le Grange D, Eisler I, Dare C, et al. Evaluation of family treatments in adolescent anorexia nervosa: a pilot study. Int J Eat Disord 1992;12(4):347–57.
19. Agras WS, Lock J, Brandt H, et al. Comparison of 2 family therapies for adolescent anorexia nervosa. JAMA Psychiatry 2014;71:1279–86.
20. Lock J, Agras WS, Bryson S, et al. A comparison of short- and long-term family therapy for adolescent anorexia nervosa. J Am Acad Child Adolesc Psychiatry 2005;44:632–9.
21. Hoste R, Labuschagne Z, Lock J, et al. Cultural variability in expressed emotion among families of adolescents with anorexia nervosa. Int J Eat Disord 2012;45: 142–5.
22. Le Grange D, Hoste R, Lock J, et al. Parental expressed emotion of adolescents with anorexia nervosa: outcome in family-based treatment. Int J Eat Disord 2011; 44(8):731–4.
23. Le Grange D, Lock J, Agras W, et al. Moderators and mediators of remission in family-based treatment and adolescent focused therapy for anorexia nervosa. Behav Res Ther 2012;50:85–92.
24. Lock J, Couturier J, Bryson S, et al. Predictors of dropout and remission in family therapy for adolescent anorexia nervosa in a randomized clinical trial. Int J Eat Disord 2006;39(8):639–47.
25. Lock J, le Grange D, Forsberg S, et al. Is family therapy useful for treating children with anorexia nervosa? results of a case series. J Am Acad Child Adolesc Psychiatry 2006;45(11):1323–8.
26. Schmidt U, Lee S, Beecham J, et al. A randomized controlled trial of family therapy and cognitive behavior therapy guided self-care for adolescents with bulimia nervosa and related conditions. Am J Psychiatry 2007;164:591–8.
27. Le Grange D, Crosby R, Rathouz P, et al. A randomized controlled comparison of family-based treatment and supportive psychotherapy for adolescent bulimia nervosa. Arch Gen Psychiatry 2007;64(9):1049–56.

28. Robin A, Siegal P, Moye A, et al. A controlled comparison of family versus individual therapy for adolescents with anorexia nervosa. J Am Acad Child Adolesc Psychiatry 1999;38(12):1482–9.
29. Eisler I, Dare C, Hodes M, et al. Family therapy for adolescent anorexia nervosa: the results of a controlled comparison of two family interventions. J Child Psychol Psychiatry 2000;41(6):727–36.
30. Lock J, Couturier J, Agras WS. Comparison of long term outcomes in adolescents with anorexia nervosa treated with family therapy. J Am Acad Child Adolesc Psychiatry 2006;45:666–72.
31. Doyle P, Le Grange D, Loeb K, et al. Early response to family-based treatment for adolescent anorexia nervosa. Int J Eat Disord 2010;43:659–62.
32. Le Grange D, Accurso E, Lock J, et al. Early weight gain predicts outcome in two treatments for adolescent anorexia nervosa. Int J Eat Disord 2014;47(2):124–9.
33. Lock J, Couturier J, Bryson S, et al. Predictors of dropout and remission in family therapy for adolescent anorexia nervosa in a randomized clinical trial. Int J Eat Disord 2006;39:639–47.
34. Le Grange D, Lock J, Agras W, et al. Moderators and mediators of remission in family-based treatment and adolescent focused therapy for anorexia nervosa. Behav Res Ther 2012;50:85–92.
35. Le Grange D, Eisler I, Dare C, et al. Family criticism and self-starvation: a study of expressed emotion. Journal of Family Therapy 1992;14:177–92.
36. Couturier J, Lock J. What constitutes remission in adolescent anorexia nervosa: a review of various conceptualizations and a quantitative analysis. Int J Eat Disord 2006;39:175–83.
37. Darcy A, Bryson S, Fitzpatrick K, et al. Do in-vivo behaviors predict early response in family-based treatment for anorexia nervosa. Behavior Research and Therapy 2013;51(11):762–6.

Family Beliefs and Intervention in Pediatric Pain Management

Christine B. Sieberg, PhD[a,b],*, Juliana Manganella, BA[a]

KEYWORDS

- Acute and chronic pain • Parent factors • Cognitive-behavioral therapy
- Acceptance and commitment-based therapy

KEY POINTS

- Acute pain will cease once the ailment has been treated or the infliction of pain has concluded.
- Chronic pain describes pain that continues once the initial stimulus is no longer present.
- Parental factors that exacerbate pain include anxiety, catastrophizing, distress, and reassurance.
- Several different measures can be used to determine parent functioning, responses, and coping as they relate to pediatric pain.
- Evidence-based parent and family interventions exist for the treatment of pediatric pain.

OVERVIEW: NATURE OF THE PROBLEM

Pain is a significant public health concern and socioeconomic burden with costs estimated to be $635 billion per year in the United States alone.[1] Pain is distinguished as either acute or chronic (although some illness conditions, such as sickle cell, can result in complex, acute, or chronic pain). This article reviews established research regarding pediatric pain and focuses on the effects of interpersonal interactions, primarily those from parents, on its expression.

This article was supported by a Boston Children's Hospital Career Development Fellowship Award to C.B. Sieberg, the Sara Page Mayo Endowment for Pediatric Pain Research and Treatment, and the Department of Anesthesiology, Perioperative and Pain Medicine at Boston Children's Hospital.

a Division of Pain Medicine, Department of Anesthesiology, Perioperative and Pain Medicine, Boston Children's Hospital, 333 Longwood Avenue, Boston, MA 02115, USA; b Department of Psychiatry, Harvard Medical School, 333 Longwood Avenue, Boston, MA 02115, USA
* Corresponding author. Pain Treatment Service, Boston Children's Hospital, 333 Longwood Avenue, 5th Floor, Boston, MA 02115.
E-mail address: christine.sieberg@childrens.harvard.edu

Child Adolesc Psychiatric Clin N Am 24 (2015) 631–645
http://dx.doi.org/10.1016/j.chc.2015.02.006
1056-4993/15/$ – see front matter © 2015 Elsevier Inc. All rights reserved.

Acute Versus Chronic Pain

The International Association for the Study of Pain defines pain as "an unpleasant sensory and emotional experience associated with actual or potential tissue damage, or described in terms of such damage."[2] Pain is classified into acute and chronic pain and is a highly subjective experience influenced by a multitude of factors. Acute pain is the umbrella term to describe the immediate onset of pain resulting from a medical event, including illness, injury, or a medical procedure. The duration of acute pain can vary, lasting from a few seconds (eg, immunization) to a few months (eg, broken bone or surgery). The primary difference between acute and chronic pain is that acute pain will cease once the ailment has been treated or the infliction of pain has concluded.[3] Managing pediatric acute pain is critical in offsetting the risk of potential development of chronic pain.

Everyone experiences acute pain. Chronic pain affects approximately 15% to 25% of children.[4,5] Much of the experimental research has been directed at acute pain. While clinical descriptions of some pain syndromes distinguish between organic and nonorganic pain, the American Pain Society maintains that this mind-body dualism conceptualization should be abandoned because all pain is associated with neurosensory changes. Even for children with an organic illness, like juvenile arthritis, the severity of pain can only be partly attributed to disease activity.[6] Musculoskeletal pain, abdominal pain, and headache are among the most common chronic pain complaints, and all are more prevalent in girls compared with boys.[7] The authors discuss here experimental research done with acute pain while realizing that chronic pain has the most damaging impact on the lives of children and families and can result in functional disability, depression, fear of pain, and pain catastrophizing.[8–12]

Summarizing research with parents and pediatric acute pain

Researchers have examined the role of parents and children in acute pain.[13–16] Many of the data cited here were generated in studies using either natural events commonly associated with pain, such as immunizations or scheduled medical procedures, or to experimental situations designed for the purpose.

Factors related to children in these studies include child distress, anxiety, and catastrophizing about the procedure.[14,17–19] Catastrophizing refers to having a response out of the range of usual expectation given the severity of the pain-generating event (making too much out of the situation). Parent factors include the parent's level of anxiety, catastrophizing, degree of reassurance given to the child, or parental distress. Family factors examined for outcomes for pediatric pain patients include aggregation of family pain complaints, parenting style, parental responses to child pain behavior, parent-child interaction, family environment, and overall family communication and functioning.[20–24]

Here are some results from these studies:

- Studies of acute pain have demonstrated that children require more restraints and express high levels of fear when parents provide reassurance during immunizations.[23,24]

- In 44 mother-child dyads, parental catastrophizing was positively related to child-reported fear of the procedural pain scenario. However, maternal catastrophizing scores did not correlate with child reports of pain.[22]
- Bearden and colleagues[14] found that parental anxiety preceding their child's immunization mediated the relationship between the child report of procedural anxiety and the child report of pain after the procedure.
- Parental distress, anxiety, and pain-specific catastrophizing have been linked to poorer outcomes, including increased pain and functional disability in children.[16,23–27]
- Parents who were trained to reassure their children during an immunization procedure were more distressed after the procedure was completed.[24]

Although it has been established that both parent distress and responses to children's pain exert significant influences on children's pain and functional outcomes, few studies have specifically addressed how these parental variables may work together. A 2010 systematic review of the literature on family factors in pediatric chronic pain yielded 16 studies that focused on associations between parent and family functioning and child pain outcomes (see Lewandowski and colleagues[21] 2010). Among those studies, researchers have found that parental response and subsequent distress in response to their child's pain contributed to higher levels of parent protective responses and feelings of helplessness and higher levels of child functional disability.[26,28] Much of the research in this realm to date has been cross-sectional, leaving open questions about whether premorbid family functioning influences pain-related disability or vice versa. Most likely, these interactions are complex and transactional.

Summarizing, interpersonal effects between parents and their children are bidirectional, with parent behaviors affecting child responses and child behaviors affecting parent responses. Most studies show that parents attempting to reassure a child about impending pain actually make the experience worse for the child.

PATIENT EVALUATION OVERVIEW: MEASURES USED TO ASSESS PARENT FACTORS IN PEDIATRIC PAIN

Blount and colleagues[16] suggest that there is not one particular assessment designed to properly gauge acute and chronic pain. They found that each tool presented individual benefits along with drawbacks. (**Table 1** contains an overview of measures.)

Interventions and Management Goals

While recognizing that much more research is needed to delineate effective treatments for both acute and chronic pediatric pain,[16,27] we can assume that types of interventions will vary with acute and chronic pain. Acute or procedural pain interventions rely primarily on parental management of their own anxiety and distress surrounding the immediate procedure through tone of voice, touch, and distraction techniques,[22,24,25,28–37] whereas chronic pain interventions require family involvement and acceptance-based strategies.[21,38,39]

Interventions for parents of children with acute pain

Children and adolescents engage in various cognitive and behavioral methods to cope with acute pain scenarios. In designing acute pain interventions, clinicians pay attention to the role played by parental preprocedural anxiety.[14] Research suggests that during medical procedures, the behavior of health care professionals is associated with the efficacy of child coping strategies, whereas parent behaviors toward their

Table 1
Assessments for parents who have a child with pain

Measure	Author, Year, Type of Pain Assessed	Validated Age Range (y)	Number of Items, Type of Report	Scoring/Scale	Example Items
OSBD-R	Elliot, Jay, & Woody, 1987; acute	2–20	8 (Behavior observation)	15-s Intervals over 4 phases (waiting, preparation, procedure, postprocedure); behaviors weighted based on intensity of distress (1–4)	Crying (1.5), screaming (4)
CAMPIS-R	Blount, Sturges, & Powers, 1990; acute	2–13	35 (Behavior observation)	6 Dimensions; categorical behavior codes; 3 child codes (coping, distress, and neutral), 3 adult codes (coping-promoting, distress, promoting, neutral)	Child humor, child crying; parent criticizing, parent directing humor toward child
BAP-PIQ	Jordan, Eccleston, McCraken, Connell, & Clinch, 2008; chronic	18+	64 Items (self-report)	1–5; Multidimensional scale	In the last 2 wk living with my child in pain I have… (eg, felt sad, not been able to get my mind off my worries, thought my child's pain would get worse, thought that I had failed my child)
PCS-P	Goubert, Eccleston, Vervoort, Jordan, & Crombaz, 2006; chronic	18+	13 Items (self-report)	1–5; Likert scale; 0 = *not at all true* to 4 = *very true*	When my child is in pain, I worry all the time about whether the pain will end. When my child is in pain, I become afraid that the pain will get worse.
Adult Response to Children's Symptoms	Van Slyke & Walker, 2006; chronic	18+	33 Items (self-report)	0 (*Never*) to 4 (*always*) Likert scale (3 subscales (*parent protectiveness, minimization of pain*)	When your child is in pain, how often do you bring your child little treats? When your child has pain, how often do you insist that your child go to school?

Abbreviations: BAP-PIQ, Bath Adolescent Pain-Parent Impact Questionnaire; CAMPIS-R, The Child-Adult Medical Procedure Interaction Scale; OSBD-R, Observational Scale of Behavior Distress-R; PCS-P, Pain Catastrophizing Scale–Parent Version.

child are correlated with child distress levels.[17,29] Parental anxiety can lead to parental distress and catastrophizing surrounding procedures, which result in higher child fear scores during acute pain procedures.[22]

It has been proposed that perhaps the reassurance behavior provided by parents during a procedure is not about what parents are saying to their children during procedural pain but how they are responding.[18,32] An example of a nonverbal parental response is the effect of touch on child distress.[32] Instrumental touch (eg, moving a child into a proper position for procedure) was positively correlated with child pain ratings during their procedure ($P<.01$), whereas parental supportive touch (eg, holding hand during a procedure) was not related to child pain levels.[32] These results suggest that parents should avoid active roles in their child's medical procedures. Additionally, McMurtry and colleagues[32] looked at how elements of speech tone, like pitch and frequency, alters the child's interpretation of reassurance during the procedure and found that children interpret parent reassurance as parent suffering and concern. Understanding how parental tone, facial expression, and verbal and nonverbal communication can influence child distress during acute pain is the first step in understanding how parents can intervene and redirect child distress during acute pain scenarios. Current research on the topic suggests parents should not try to help with the procedure (eg, holding a child down) and, instead, they should show support through both verbal and nonverbal statements, by paying close attention to the tone and pitch of their communication.[31,32] Additionally, there are behavioral techniques that parents can engage in, with the hopes of relieving some of their child's distress.

Various researchers have examined the bidirectional impact that exists between parent behavior and cognitions surrounding their child's medical procedures and how it impacts both parent and child pain perceptions and distress.[13,28,29,33] Distraction is a commonly studied behavioral technique used during medical procedures or acute pain interventions.[13,17,34–36] Distraction techniques include having an adult change the subject to get the child's mind off the procedure, and using age appropriate toys or videos to redirect the attention of the child. The effects of nurse, parent, and child led distraction have each been examined.[13,17,36] The findings support the idea that using a distraction technique alleviates some amount of distress in parents and infants, children, and adolescents compared with when parents interact in a usual manner.[28] In particular, one study found that daughters whose mothers reacted in a pain-reducing manner (eg, distraction techniques) reported less pain intensity during a cold-pressor task (experimental pain paradigm) than daughters in the control group.[37] This idea was further supported in a study of nurse-led distraction during infant immunizations. The infants in the distraction group exhibited less distress than the infants in the normative care group.[28] A systematic review[15] of psychological interventions for procedural pain categorized 7 different procedural pain interventions and examined the ways in which these interventions were effective. In general, parent-led distractions (eg, use of toys, modeling, verbal distraction) were found to be effective in reducing parental distress and anxiety about the procedure; but the findings were ambivalent as to whether distraction actually altered child pain perceptions.[15] This finding suggests that reminding parents to be calm and supportive of their child during procedures is as effective as using other distraction techniques.

Interventions for parents of children with chronic pain

Given the significant impact of parent factors on pediatric chronic pain outcomes, parent involvement in the treatment of complex pediatric pain is essential. Although more studies of family based interventions in pediatric pain are needed, some important research has been conducted in the area of recurrent and/or functional abdominal pain as well as in pain rehabilitation.

Sanders and colleagues[40] examined the comparative efficacy of a cognitive-behavioral (cognitive-behavioral therapy [CBT]) family based intervention and standard pediatric care for children experiencing recurrent (also referred to as *functional*) abdominal pain (RAP). Forty-four children with RAP aged 7 to 14 years were randomized into one of 2 groups (cognitive-behavioral family or pediatric care). All children used a visual analog scale to record pain intensity. The cognitive-behavioral family component consisted of 6 sessions that included psychoeducation about RAP, contingency management training for parents, and self-management strategy training for children. Children in the standard pediatric care treatment met regularly with their pediatrician who provided reassurance and support as well as instructing children that they must cope with their pain but did not provide specific coping skills. Children in the treatment group were found to have fewer pain symptoms and less pain intensity at after treatment and at the 6- and 12-month follow-up.

Additionally, Robins and colleagues[41] compared the combination of standard medical care and short-term cognitive-behavioral family treatment (n = 40) versus standard medical care alone (n = 29) for the treatment of RAP. The intervention consisted of presenting a model of recurrent pain to children and parents, instructing children in the active management of pain episodes, modeling and practicing pain management techniques, and assisting parents in developing more adaptive responses to their child's pain. Results indicated that children and parents participating in the combined intervention reported significantly less child- and parent-reported child abdominal pain and fewer school absences than children receiving only standard medical care immediately following the intervention and up to 1 year following the study entry.

Sieberg and colleagues[12] conducted a multiple-baseline across participants (n = 8 families) design using repeated measures of anxiety and pain to examine the utility of a CBT and a treatment that combined both CBT and family based approaches in a community sample of children with comorbid anxiety and RAP. Via a diagnostic structured interview assessing anxiety (Anxiety Disorders Interview Schedule[42]), children had to meet the criteria for an anxiety disorder at baseline. Specifically, the family based condition combined the CBT protocol[43] with an intervention designed to improve parent-child interaction as well as parental responses to child pain. The family component of this condition was based on Beardslee and colleagues'[44] Family Based Preventive Intervention, an empirically supported manualized treatment developed originally for the prevention of depressive symptoms in children of depressed parents. Clinical significance analyses indicate that both treatment conditions were effective at reducing anxiety and abdominal pain. Although family based CBT holds promise for the treatment of RAP, aside from this study, there are no other empirically based studies assessing family based therapies for the treatment of RAP *and* anxiety. Including parents in learning CBT strategies with their child, while also focusing on family functioning, is an important future direction for randomized clinical trials (**Figs. 1** and **2**).

TREATMENT RESISTANCE AND COMPLICATIONS

When outpatient modalities are not sufficient, an intensive treatment approach, such as a partial hospital or comprehensive rehabilitation program, may be warranted. Multidisciplinary and interdisciplinary day hospital programs are gaining attention as a necessary treatment option for pediatric complex chronic pain, and these programs

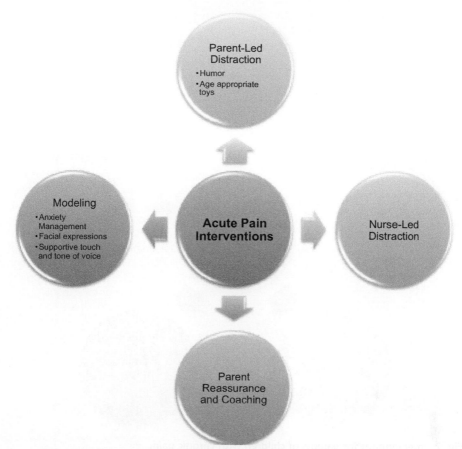

Fig. 1. Interventions for parents with a child undergoing procedural pain.

require parental involvement for admission. Early studies show that parents whose children are enrolled in these intensive programs improve in their perception of their child's functional disability as well as have improved scores for their own anxiety, depression, and parental stress.[45] Furthermore, parents of children enrolled in these programs have been shown to be more willing to allow their child to adopt a self-management approach to pain. They also reported reductions in their perceptions of their child's fear of pain with treatment.[46] Unfortunately, although this treatment approach is gaining momentum, few of these programs exist worldwide.

Treatment goals for parents enrolled in such programs typically include:

- Addressing parental responses to pain
- Helping parents to foster self-management of pain within their child
- Addressing family dynamics and interactions around pain

The day treatment model provides a higher intensity of care and treatment coordination than can be afforded through outpatient services while providing patients opportunities to rehearse the skills they are learning during nontreatment hours. Interventions in these programs often include parent groups, individual parent support

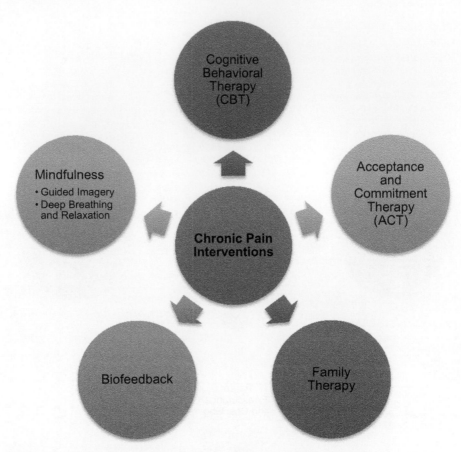

Fig. 2. Interventions for parents of children with chronic pain.

and counseling, family therapy, and parent observation of treatment modalities, including physical and occupational therapy. For many parents enrolled in these programs, learning not to protect their child from pain feels counterintuitive.

The following case study highlights the role of cognitive-behavioral family therapy in conjunction with alternative therapeutic treatment modalities including the following:

- Biofeedback is a noninvasive technique, which monitors the body's physiologic sensations through electrical sensors. The sensors provide patients information about their bodily functioning through a sound or visual cue, with the goal of fostering patients' awareness of their physiologic reactions and subsequent behavior.
- Deep breathing, relaxation, and guided imagery is a technique used to treat ailments ranging from anxiety to pain through the foundations of the mind-body connection, altered state, and locus of control. Self-imagery can be engaged in verbally or visually through the use of a script or image.
- Behavior plans are utilized to target problematic pain behaviors (eg, not attending school) that are impacting functioning. Behavior plans rely on positive reinforcement to achieve behavior change.

CLINICAL EXAMPLE 1

Anna (All names and identifying information have been changed.), an 8-year-old girl, presented to the Pain Service with a recent onset of neuropathic pain in her right lower leg that impacted her gait and that resulted in significant behavioral regression, mood lability, separation anxiety, and sleep difficulties. Given the impact her pain and emotions were having on her functioning (eg, missing school, not able to leave her mother), Anna was admitted to a day hospital for children with complex chronic pain. Anna and her parents participated in twice-weekly family CBT sessions for 3 weeks. During these sessions, it was apparent that Anna's parents had drastically different responses to Anna's pain behaviors. Her mother was observed allowing her daughter to avoid pain-provoking activities. She also interacted with Anna as if she was much younger (eg, talking to her in baby talk) and provided positive attention to Anna (eg, buying her presents) when Anna was in pain. Her father tended to ignore Anna's behaviors but was also distant as if he wanted to avoid the problem. Parent sessions focused on having parents communicate about their different responses and problem solving around more appropriate responses to Anna's pain, such as ignoring pain behaviors and providing praise when Anna engaged in an age-appropriate task (eg, doing homework). Given Anna's young age, the parents also participated in family based physical and occupational therapy sessions with a psychologist present. These sessions focused on having the psychologist provide feedback in the moment regarding parent-child interactions around pain. Family CBT sessions also included constructing numerous behavioral plans to promote positive, active coping as well as teaching biobehavioral strategies for pain management, such as deep breathing, relaxation, biofeedback, and guided self-imagery. At the end of 3 weeks, Anna was walking with an even gait, displaying developmentally appropriate behavior, and was engaged in active coping skills. Her mother stated that she wanted to become a support for other parents dealing with children with chronic pain conditions. Anna successfully returned to school. At 1 year after discharge, gains were maintained and overall Anna was functioning well.

Adopting an acceptance-based treatment approach to family therapy, especially by exploring values, can also be effective. These techniques can foster a shift in the family's perspective from paying attention to illness and pain to rewarding functioning. This type of intensive treatment model can be highly effective at altering a family's shared belief system around pain and illness and decreasing parents' distress and protective responses to their children, thus, fostering more adaptive coping in all family members.

The following clinical example incorporates the model of acceptance and commitment therapy (ACT).[47,48] The goals of ACT are as follows:

- Unpack and decipher individual cognitions surrounding communication
- Recognize thoughts and emotions without judgment with the goal of becoming self-aware
- Set personal goals based on individual values

CLINICAL EXAMPLE 2

Emily, a 16-year-old girl, presented to the Pediatric Headache Program with a 2-year history of intermittent and predominantly tension-type headaches as well as migraines secondary to a viral infection. Complicating her presentation was a longstanding history of attention-deficit/hyperactivity disorder (ADHD), inattentive subtype, anxiety, and depression since 10 years of age. Emily also had a trauma history. Since the onset of her pain, Emily had had significant functional disability (eg, school avoidance, quitting softball). Notable family history included anxiety, depression, substance abuse, and borderline personality disorder. Emily had seen more than 5 different therapists in the past for her multiple mental health issues; however, the coping skills she had previously learned for her anxiety and depression were not helpful for her pain. Despite trying numerous medications, injections, and physical therapy, pain and disability persisted and Emily was referred for pain-focused psychology.

When Emily presented to therapy, she stated, "With the migraines, sometimes they prohibit me from doing what I want to do. The frustration that comes along with this also lowers my self-esteem. The depression and headaches are a vicious cycle; I'm most often dealing with one or the other, and sometimes both."

Emily's therapeutic course was long and difficult. She was seen for 88 sessions. It became apparent during treatment that Emily required a different orientation from CBT or biofeedback. She was keenly aware that her mental health and pain issues were longstanding, and she was not sure they would ever change. Treatment shifted focus to an acceptance orientation. Specifically, mindfulness strategies were used, and treatment focused on values clarification in order to enhance psychological flexibility and help target avoidance-based behavior that can interfere with quality of life and values-based living. For Emily, this included doing well in school, taking care of her nieces, and eventually becoming a doctor so she could help others. To accomplish this, Emily had to be willing to experience distressing physical sensations, emotions, and thoughts that interfered with her ability to alter dysfunctional behavior. Importantly, in order to accomplish this, Emily's mother also had to be willing to allow her daughter to experience distress.

She had a strong, dependent relationship with her mother. Although her mother sometimes joined the sessions, Emily's goal became coming to the sessions alone and being an advocate for herself. To this end, Emily's mother was typically seen at the end of each session for parenting work. Emily's mother wanted a quick fix for Emily and could not understand the shift in therapy to an ACT approach. At one point, she threatened to take Emily out of therapy if Emily experienced any type of distress. She initially refused to think that her daughter would ever have to cope with long-term pain, depression, or anxiety. Parent sessions focused on providing psychoeducation on the ACT model as well as exploring the mother's own values as well as values she held for her daughter. She said that she wanted Emily to be able to reintegrate back to school and eventually be able to move out of the home to attend college. Having Emily and her mother engage in ACT was effective. Emily was gradually able to get back to school and eventually graduated among the top of her class before enrolling in a nationally ranked university. Today she still experiences anxiety, panic attacks, and depression but rarely has headaches and has not had any interventional injections in more than 2 years.

Outpatient therapy can often be effective, but sometimes complicated family dynamics and impaired family functioning requires a more intensive treatment approach. The following clinical example highlights how family therapy sessions in the context of intensive rehabilitation can be used to identify the maladaptive dynamics that exist within the family system. Specifically this case uses:

- Family systems therapy and parent-based intervention
- Incorporating dual-parent functioning in child's treatment
- Family dynamics and communication

CLINICAL EXAMPLE 3

Jack, a 15-year-old boy, presented to the Pain Service with a 2-year history of postural orthostatic tachycardia syndrome (POTS) and comorbid anxiety, obsessive-compulsive disorder, and ADHD, inattentive subtype. His POTS symptoms also included diffuse body pain and headaches. He described his pain as "severe enough to keep me from doing anything," which was accurate as he had not attended school in 2 years and rarely left home. He reported, "I don't have the strength to get to the bathroom." His sister also had a longstanding history of chronic pain. Because of Jack's level of disability, he was admitted to the same program as Anna (described earlier). His family psychology sessions were different from Anna's. There was a strong pattern of modeling and reinforcement of pain and illness behaviors in the family. His mother had quit her job to remain at home with her children after they became sick.

During family sessions, the mother was highly protective of Jack and constantly asked him if he needed to lie down or needed food. Jack often turned to his father before responding to questions. The treatment team learned about developmentally inappropriate interactions, such as cosleeping at home and observed disproportionate amounts of hugging and kissing during psychology sessions. Family sessions focused on addressing family dynamics and interactions around pain. The authors came to understand that father felt left out of the family unit. He revealed that since his 2 children had developed POTS and diffuse body pain, he felt that he did not exist. The family was previously active and particularly enjoyed hiking and rock climbing but no longer left home. He expressed that he felt forgotten; he was not even able to sleep with his wife who was cosleeping with her 2 adolescent children. Family sessions focused on giving the father a voice to express these feelings as well as problem solving how to promote functioning and shift the identity of the family from one of illness and disability to one of functioning and wellness. The authors asked the parents to write down all the ways in which the family had changed, everything from not leaving home and cosleeping to little things like who clears the table after dinner and all the hobbies the mother and father are no longer engaged in. They then shared this with each other, which was the catalyst for change. The mother acknowledged that she had no idea how much had changed within the family. The authors also addressed some longer-standing family interaction patterns influencing the pain experience, such as stubborn, argumentative, and rigid personality styles.

After a 5-week admission, Jack no longer had POTS symptoms and was discharged to school. Four months after discharge, Jack was back at school full-time and the family was exercising and rock climbing together, gains that were maintained at the 1-year follow-up.

NEW CLINICAL DIRECTIONS

The authors spend much of the early part of this article describing how parents can make their children's acute pain worse through their anxiety, or attempts at reassurance, and even suggest they play a minimal role during pediatric procedures. Conversely, with chronic pain, family involvement is often crucial for improvement to take place. A Cochrane Review supports this position by concluding there is good efficacy for the inclusion of parents in psychological therapies aimed at pain reduction and management for children with painful conditions.[49]

Most clinical interventions for parents of children with chronic pain are imbedded within child-focused interventions and are psychoeducational and behaviorally based as a way to augment the child's ability to manage and cope with pain.[41,45,50] One recent study implemented a pilot parent-only art-therapy group curriculum for 53 parents of children enrolled in an intensive day hospital pediatric pain rehabilitation program.[51] The group art-therapy intervention was designed specifically to target the struggles of parents of children with chronic pain (seeking support, managing feelings of burden, helplessness, isolation, fear, and lack of time for self). This parent-only art group is the first of its kind and represents an innovative approach to addressing the needs of parents in this treatment setting. Additionally, the modules developed for this intervention were intended to help parents reflect on their *own* experiences, feelings, sacrifices, and difficulties since the onset of their child's pain, as opposed to asking the parents to retell their child's history. In this way, parents were encouraged to use their unique voice and narrate their own story. The pilot study evaluated parents' initial responses to the art-therapy groups, measured by perceived satisfaction and helpfulness. Results indicated that parents enjoyed participating in the group, agreed that they would try art therapy again, and found it to be a helpful, supportive, and validating experience.[51] More interventions such as these are warranted for the interdisciplinary treatment of complex pain.

SUMMARY

Parents of children undergoing medical procedures and with chronic pain have their own unique needs, separate from those of their children, which can still impact their child's pain experience and rehabilitation process. As discussed earlier, evidence of high levels of distress experienced by parents of children with chronic pain is well documented[52,53] as is recognition of their key role in how their child copes with and recovers from pain.[39]

Understanding the child and his or her pain experience in the context of the family is the key for addressing this widespread and impactful aspect of childhood. Future research should aim to include fathers, as most pediatric research typically focuses on mothers. This point is especially important given the recent findings that demonstrate differences in catastrophizing between mothers and fathers.[54] Siblings of children with pain are also a neglected area of research and warrant further investigation and inclusion of them into family based treatments for pediatric pain.

REFERENCES

1. Gaskin D, Richard P. The economic costs of pain in the US. J Pain 2012;13(8): 715.
2. IASP taxonomy. Updated 2012. Available at: http://www.iasp-pain.org/. Accessed July 26, 2014.
3. American Academy of Pediatrics. Committee on psychosocial aspects of child and family health, task force on pain in infants, children, and adolescents. The assessment and management of acute pain in infants, children, and adolescents. Pediatrics 2001;108(3):793–7.
4. Goodman JE, McGrath PJ. The epidemiology of pain in children and adolescents: a review. Pain 1991;46(3):247–64.
5. Roth-Isigkeit A, Thyen U, Stoven H, et al. Pain among children and adolescents: restrictions in daily living and triggering factors. Pediatrics 2005;115(2):152–62.
6. Malleson PN, Clinch J. Pain syndromes in children. Curr Opin Pharmacol 2003; 15:572–80.
7. King S, Chambers CT, Huguet A, et al. The epidemiology of chronic pain in children and adolescents revisited: a systematic review. Pain 2011;152:2729–38.
8. Dorn LD, Campo JC, Thato S, et al. Psychological comorbidity and stress reactivity in children and adolescents with recurrent abdominal pain and anxiety disorders. J Am Acad Child Adolesc Psychiatry 2003;42(1):66–75.
9. Campo JV, Bridge J, Ehmann M, et al. Recurrent abdominal pain, anxiety, and depression in primary care. Pediatrics 2004;113(4):817.
10. Eccleston C, Crombez G, Scotford A, et al. Adolescent chronic pain: patterns and predictors of emotional distress in adolescents with chronic pain and their parents. Pain 2004;108:221–9.
11. Quartana PJ, Campbell CM, Edwards RR. Pain catastrophizing: a critical review. Expert Rev Neurother 2009;9:745–58.
12. Sieberg CB, Flannery-Schroeder E, Plante W. Children with co-morbid recurrent abdominal pain and anxiety disorders: results from a multiple-baseline pilot study. J Child Health Care 2011;15(2):126–39.
13. Cramer-Berness LJ, Friedman AG. Behavioral interventions for infant immunizations. Child Health Care 2005;34:95–111.
14. Bearden DJ, Feinstein A, Cohen LL. The influence of parent preprocedural anxiety on child procedural pain: mediation by child procedural anxiety. J Pediatr Psychol 2012;37:680–6.

15. Chambers CT, Taddio A, Uman LS, et al. Psychological interventions for reducing pain and distress during routine childhood immunizations: a systematic review. Clin Ther 2009;31:S77–102.
16. Blount RL, Zempsky WT, Jaaniste T, et al. Management of pediatric pain and distress due to medical procedures. In: Roberts MC, Steele RG, editors. Handbook of pediatric psychology, Vol. 4. New York: Guilford Press; 2009. p. 171–88.
17. Cohen LL, Bernard RS, Greco LA, et al. A child-focused intervention for coping with procedural pain: are parent and nurse coaches necessary? J Pediatr Psychol 2002;28:749–57.
18. McMurtry CM, McGrath PJ, Chambers CT. Reassurance can hurt: parental behavior and painful medical procedures. J Pediatr 2006;148:560–1.
19. Bernard RS, Cohen LL. Parent anxiety and infant pain during pediatric immunizations. J Clin Psychol Med Settings 2006;13:285–90.
20. Palermo TM, Chambers CT. Parent and family factors in pediatric chronic pain and disability: an integrative approach. J Pain 2005;119:1–4.
21. Lewandowski AS, Palermo TM, Stinson JN, et al. Systematic review of family functioning in families of children and adolescents with chronic pain. J Pain 2010;11: 1027–38.
22. Vervoort T, Goubert L, Vandenbossche H, et al. Child's and parent's catastrophizing about pain is associated with procedural fear in children: a study in children with diabetes and their mothers. Psychol Rep 2011;109:879–95.
23. Blount RL, Bunke V, Cohen LL, et al. The child-adult medical procedure interaction scale-short form (CAMPIS-SF): validation of a rating scale for children's and adults' behaviors during painful medical procedures. J Pain Symptom Manage 2001;22:591–9.
24. Manimala MR, Blount RL, Cohen LL. The effects of parental reassurance versus distraction on child distress and coping during immunizations. Child Health Care 2000;29:161–77.
25. Goubert L, Craig KD, Vervoort T, et al. Facing others in pain: the effects of empathy. Pain 2005;118:285–8.
26. Caes L, Vervoort T, Eccleston C, et al. Parental catastrophizing about child's pain and its relationship with activity restriction: the mediating role of parental distress. Pain 2011;152:212–22.
27. Kazak AE, Simms S, Rourke MT. Family systems practice in pediatric psychology. J Pediatr Psychol 2002;27:133–43.
28. Cohen LL, MacLaren JE, Fortson BL, et al. Randomized clinical trial of distraction for infant immunization pain. Pain 2006;125:165–71.
29. Mahoney L, Ayers S, Seddon P. The association between parent's and healthcare professional's behavior and children's coping and distress during venepuncture. J Pediatr Psychol 2010;35:985–95.
30. McMurtry MC. Pediatric needle procedures: parent–child interactions, child fear, and evidence-based treatment. Can Psychol 2013;54:75–9.
31. Peterson AM, Cline RJW, Foster TS, et al. Parents' interpersonal distance and touch behavior and child pain and distress during painful pediatric oncology procedures. J Nonverbal Behav 2007;31:71–97.
32. McMurtry MC, McGrath PJ, Asp E, et al. Parental reassurance and pediatric procedural pain: a linguistic description. J Pain 2007;8:95–101.
33. Blount RL, Piira T, Cohen LL. Management of pediatric pain and distress due to medical procedures. In: Roberts MC, editor. Handbook of pediatric psychology, Vol. 3. New York: Guildford Press; 2003. p. 216–33.

34. Cassidy KL, Reid GJ, McGrath PJ, et al. Watch needle, watch TV: audiovisual distraction in preschool immunization. Pain Med 2002;3:108–18.
35. Walker LS, Williams SE, Smith CA, et al. Parent attention versus distraction: impact on symptom complaints by children with and without functional abdominal pain. Pain 2006;122:43–52.
36. Inal S, Kelleci M. Distracting children during blood draw: looking through distraction cards is effective in pain relief of children during blood draw. Int J Nurs Stud 2012;18:210–9.
37. Chambers CT, Craig KD, Bennett SM. The impact of maternal behavior on children's pain experiences: an experimental analysis. J Pediatr Psychol 2002;27: 293–301.
38. Palermo TM, Eccleston C, Lewandowski AS, et al. Randomized controlled trials of psychological therapies for management of chronic pain in children and adolescents: an updated meta-analytic review. Pain 2010;148(3):387–97.
39. Vowles KE, Cohen LL, McCracken LM, et al. Disentangling the complex relations among caregiver and adolescent responses to adolescent chronic pain. Pain 2010;151:680–6.
40. Sanders MR, Shepherd RW, Cleghorn G, et al. The treatment of recurrent abdominal pain in children: a controlled comparison of cognitive-behavioral family intervention and standard pediatric care. J Consult Clin Psychol 1994;62(2):306–14.
41. Robins P, Smith SB, Gluttin J, et al. A randomized controlled trial of a cognitive-behavioral family intervention for recurrent abdominal pain. J Pediatr Psychol 2005;30:397–408.
42. Silverman WK, Saavedra LM, Pina AA. Test retest reliability of anxiety symptoms and diagnoses with the anxiety disorders interview schedule for DSM-IV: child and parent versions. J Am Acad Child Adolesc Psychiatry 2001;40:937–44.
43. Savedra MC, Holzemer WL, Tesler MD, et al. Assessment of postoperation pain in children and adolescents using the adolescent pediatric pain tool. Nurs Res 1993;42(1):5–9.
44. Beardslee WR, Gladstone TR, Wright EJ, et al. A family based approach to the prevention of depressive symptoms in children at risk: evidence of parental and child change. Pediatrics 2003;112:e119–31.
45. Eccleston C, Malleson PN, Clinch J, et al. Chronic pain in adolescents: evaluation of a programme of interdisciplinary cognitive behaviour therapy. Arch Dis Child 2003;88:881–5.
46. Logan DE, Conroy C, Sieberg CB, et al. Changes in willingness to self-manage pain among children and adolescents and their parents enrolled in an intensive interdisciplinary pediatric pain treatment program. Pain 2012;153(9):1863–70.
47. Hayes SC, Pistorello J, Levin ME. Acceptance and commitment therapy as a unified model of behavior change. Couns Psychol 2012;976–1002.
48. McCracken LM, Vowles KE. Acceptance and commitment therapy and mindfulness for chronic pain: model, process, and progress. Am Psychol 2014;69: 178–87.
49. Eccleston C, Palermo TM, Fisher E, et al. Psychological interventions for parents of children and adolescents with chronic illness. Cochrane Database Syst Rev 2012;(8):CD009660.
50. Palermo TM, Wilson AC, Peters M, et al. Randomized controlled trial of an internet-delivered family cognitive–behavioral therapy intervention for children and adolescents with chronic pain. Pain 2009;146:205–13.
51. Pielech M, Sieberg CB, Simons LE. Connecting parents of children with chronic pain through art therapy. Clin Pract Pediatr Psychol 2013;1(3):214–26.

52. Palermo TM, Putnam J, Armstrong G, et al. Adolescent autonomy and family functioning are associated with headache related disability. Clin J Pain 2007; 23:458–65.

53. Logan DE, Scharff L. Relationships between family and parent characteristics and functional abilities in children with recurrent pain syndromes: an investigation of moderating effects on the pathway from pain to disability. J Pediatr 2005;30(8): 698–707.

54. Hechler T, Vervoort T, Hamann M, et al. Parental catastrophizing about their child's chronic pain: are mothers and fathers different? Eur J Pain 2011;15(5):515.

Index

Note: Page numbers of article titles are in **boldface** type.

A

Child Adolesc Psychiatric Clin N Am 24 (2015) 647–658
http://dx.doi.org/10.1016/S1056-4993(15)00035-8
1056-4993/15/$ – see front matter © 2015 Elsevier Inc. All rights reserved.

childpsych.theclinics.com

Moving?

Make sure your subscription moves with you!

To notify us of your new address, find your **Clinics Account Number** (located on your mailing label above your name), and contact customer service at:

Email: journalscustomerservice-usa@elsevier.com

800-654-2452 (subscribers in the U.S. & Canada)
314-447-8871 (subscribers outside of the U.S. & Canada)

Fax number: 314-447-8029

Elsevier Health Sciences Division
Subscription Customer Service
3251 Riverport Lane
Maryland Heights, MO 63043

*To ensure uninterrupted delivery of your subscription, please notify us at least 4 weeks in advance of move.

Printed and bound by CPI Group (UK) Ltd, Croydon, CR0 4YY
03/10/2024
01040465-0004